# Talking Back

# Talking Back

## How to Overcome Chronic Back Pain and Rebuild Your Life

Rowland G. Hazard, MD

ROWMAN & LITTLEFIELD
Lanham · Boulder · New York · London

The ideas and strategies in this book are not meant to substitute for the care and guidance of a skilled and trusted personal physician. The author recommends that readers begin their recovery programs by reviewing their health and treatment plans for safety and guidance with their doctor. The author and publisher disclaim any liability for health outcomes generated by following the suggestions in this book.

Published by Rowman & Littlefield
An imprint of The Rowman & Littlefield Publishing Group, Inc.
4501 Forbes Boulevard, Suite 200, Lanham, Maryland 20706
www.rowman.com

6 Tinworth Street, London SE11 5AL, United Kingdom

British Library Cataloguing in Publication Information Available

**Library of Congress Cataloging-in-Publication Data**

Names: Hazard, Rowland, 1949– author.
Title: Talking back : how to overcome chronic back pain and rebuild your life / Rowland G. Hazard, MD.
Description: Lanham : Rowman & Littlefield, [2021] | Includes index. | Summary: "Back pain afflicts more than 3 in 4 adults and costs Americans over $100 billion every year. While most people recover quickly, the disabilities suffered by people who don't generate the vast majority of the costs and heartache. Talking Back offers people disabled by chronic back pain personal strategies for recovering active lives and wellness" — Provided by publisher.
Identifiers: LCCN 2020047797 (print) | LCCN 2020047798 (ebook) | ISBN 9781538146651 (cloth) | ISBN 9781538146668 (ebook)
Subjects: LCSH: Backache—Popular works. | Chronic diseases—Popular works. | Communication in medicine.
Classification: LCC RD771.B217 H39 2021 (print) | LCC RD771.B217 (ebook) | DDC 617.5/64—dc23
LC record available at https://lccn.loc.gov/2020047797
LC ebook record available at https://lccn.loc.gov/2020047798

*To*
*Bobbie Lanahan*

# Contents

# Preface

$\mathcal{L}$ike three out of four Americans, you have probably suffered through an attack of back pain. Surely, you know someone who has. Chances are 9 out of 10 that the episode resolved, with or without any treatment. If so, you don't need to read this book.

*Talking Back* is for the millions of "1 out of 10s" who, despite their best efforts to get rid of their pain, continue to suffer for months and even for many years. Worse than that, their pain disables them. They not only hurt every day; they also can't do the most meaningful things in life. Work, play, and even essential daily activities are limited or impossible.

Americans spend more than $100 billion every year on back pain. You have no doubt been touched in some way by the enormous and growing economic burden of health care. So, you might expect that tests and treatments for back pain account for the billions spent. You would be wrong. The vast majority of the money covers the costs of disability, not medical care.

Rather than proposing novel interventions to cure back pain, *Talking Back* aims to help people disabled by chronic pain to get their lives back on track. The lessons you are about to learn are drawn from my conversations with small groups of more than 3,000 pain-disabled participants in rehabilitation centers known as functional restoration programs (FRPs). These programs were conducted at the University of Vermont between 1986 and 2000 and subsequently at the Dartmouth-Hitchcock Medical Center in New Hampshire from 2002 through my retirement in 2018.

Three groups of people made *Talking Back* possible, and I want to thank them. First, I am deeply indebted to my early orthopedic teachers and mentors. John Frymoyer, MD, my chairman at the University of Vermont, supported my 1985 fellowship at the University of Texas Health Science Center in Dallas, where Tom Mayer, MD, and Vert Mooney, MD, introduced me to the principles of functional restoration. I also want to thank my fellow members of the International Society for the Study of the Lumbar Spine for their collegial questioning and encouragement over the years.

More than 50 health caretakers served with me in FRPs at the University of Vermont and Dartmouth. Nurses, physical and occupational therapists and their assistants, trainers, psychologists, caseworkers, and office staff worked together in multidisciplinary teams like I had never seen before. While I am grateful for their service and spirit, my gratitude pales before the thanks expressed by the thousands of patients they have helped get back on their feet.

Most important, I want to thank the patients who entrusted their care to me and the FRP teams. Many of these people had to overcome doubts about medical providers, born out of previous encounters, in order to let down their defenses and share their truths with us and with each other. I applaud their courage.

Each of the seven chapters you are about to read is drawn from small-group discussions that evolved over the years in FRP classrooms. Beginning as authoritarian lectures about things we medical "experts" thought everyone should know, they became conversations between patients and staff in which we learned together what works and what doesn't work for people disabled by chronic back pain. I have done my best to distill their wisdom for you, and I hope their collective voice helps you along your way to wellness.

# • 1 •

# No One Knows Your Pain
# the Way That You Do

$\mathcal{I}$magine that you are sitting at a conference table with six other people. You have been told that they have all suffered from back pain for at least 3 months, most of them for a matter of years. You will learn that these men and women come from various walks of life, but they have in common the reason they are there: pain severely limits their work, play, or activities of daily living. They are disabled, though you would not know that by looking at them. They have had all kinds of tests and imaging. They have "tried everything" to fix their pain, including injections, pills, surgeries, manipulation, acupuncture, hanging upside down, exercise, rest—you name it. Strangers who have only just met, they are getting started in an intensive all-day, 3-week rehabilitation experience called the functional restoration program (FRP).

## ROBERTA

First, meet Roberta, sitting on your right; more like perching on the edge of her seat. She gets up from time to time to stand and lean forward, supporting herself with her elbows on the back of her chair. You struggle with whether to ask her if there is anything you can do for her, but you don't. No one else does, and you are not sure yet how to behave in this group. Hold on to that uncertainty. You will see how important it is in a few minutes.

Roberta is a wispy-thin 35-year-old former loan officer with a pink streak in her platinum hair and not enough mascara to hide the

1

depression in her eyes. You will learn that she is a single mother of four school-age kids and that she had always depended on exercise to curb her anxiety and dark moods. She never had what you would call an injury, but when she developed back pain, she couldn't tolerate long hours of desk work. She lost her job at the bank and, on a neighbor's advice, stopped going to the gym. After 2 years of tests and treatments of all sorts, her savings dwindled. She told the kids they would have to move to an apartment in a "more affordable" town. She broke down in her doctor's office, finally admitting to another person her hopelessness and fear of destitution. Little comfort and no plan came from the response, "I'm sorry, but we just don't know what's wrong with you."

A large whiteboard hangs on the wall with colored markers in the tray. I walk in and introduce myself. Taking off my hospital coat and MD badge, I sit down and explain that this is my favorite part of the program. I get to put aside my doctor role and all the expectations that may go with it. My plan is to share with these patients ideas that have come from meeting with groups like theirs over many years. Most of the ideas come from stories of previous FRP patients; the rest are carefully researched answers to their questions. Many of the ideas would surely raise the eyebrows of established medical practitioners.

Why do I trust in these ideas? Because they come from so many different people with such a variety of clinical and personal problems, consistently asking the same questions and reaching the same conclusions. Over the years, their stories and questions have fashioned these themes of personal wisdom like beating pieces of metal into practical tools.

To clarify who has the most firsthand experience with pain, I ask how long each person has had his or her current problem. The answers typically range from 6 months to 20 years, the average total for the group almost always topping 50 years. Fifty years! That is far longer than my 30 years of taking care of people in pain. So rather than me lecturing them on what is wrong with them and how to solve all their problems, it makes sense to pool our knowledge and to address together their personal situations and questions.

## PAIN TALK

Stepping up to the board, I ask what words they have actually used to talk to other people about their pain. I write the words on the board in three columns. Figure 1.1 shows a typical list. I try to give everyone plenty of time, especially the apparently shyer members. Often, they encourage each other, and there are bursts of approval and recognition in response to the words they use in common, but there is a certain tension brewing. When the group runs out of words, there always comes a heavy silence. I let it linger long enough so that the group clearly becomes uncomfortable.

---

**WORDS YOU HAVE USED TO TALK ABOUT YOUR PAIN**

| | | |
|---|---|---|
| Achy | Wicked | Stopped Trying |
| Dull | Wipes Me Out | Never Mind |
| Sharp | Terrible | Gave Up |
| Burning | Excruciating | Hate Talking About It |
| Numby | Toothache | Lonely |
| Pinching | !!#@!!^))!! | |
| Stabbing | Knife In My Back | |
| | 0 – 10 | |

---

**Figure 1.1.**

"What is going on here? Fifty years, and this is all you got?" Then the emotions roll out, reflecting the frustration and resignation in column 3 on the right. It is unusual not to have both tears and expletives. To everyone, the most striking point made by the list is how short it is and how members of the group vary widely in the number and complexity of their personal terms. This is new territory for all. Almost none of them has ever discussed the challenge of talking about their pain and feeling so not heard.

When I ask the group about the purpose of the words in column 1, they respond that these are describing the quality of their pain. So why would you bother to describe how your pain feels to another person? In general, you want the other person to understand what is wrong with you, but that understanding depends on who that person is in crucial ways. First, if the person is a family member or acquaintance without medical training, you hope that he or she will grasp the nature of your pain so that he or she will know how to behave around you. If you have cancer or another serious disease, sympathy and physical assistance might be appropriate. If it's just a strain and quick recovery is expected, the person might simply be encouraging or dismissive. Ever come home from an emergency room visit and have to tell someone that the pain that was severe enough to call an ambulance was "just a strain"? Try that for an exercise in humiliation. Guess what kind of reaction you will get from your boss if the back pain that has kept you out of work for 6 weeks is "nothing serious," according to the doctor.

How successful has the group been in conveying the nature of their pain to laypeople? This question always produces reports and recollections of deep frustration, even anger. The inability of family members to appreciate the nature of a person's daily suffering from these descriptive words is distressing. However, medical providers frequently prove even more problematic. As we will see in chapter 3, patients with chronic back pain rarely feel that their provider really understands what is causing their pain well enough to provide appropriate and effective care. No wonder so many people with chronic back pain feel misunderstood by and isolated from the people who matter most to them.

> Roberta: "I feel so bad for my kids. They just can't understand how much my back hurts. I know they love me, but it seems like they either feel sorry for me or they're mad at me for not doing things with them. My doctor is even worse. She doesn't even examine me. She just types on her computer until I'm done talking, which I don't do much anymore. What's the use?"

## HOW MUCH DOES IT HURT?

Moving over to the words in column 2, the group realizes that they are trying to express the severity of the pain. Some words do this directly ("really bad") and others by describing the emotional results of the pain ("sucks the spirit out of you"). Here the individuals in the group vary widely in their ability to find expressive words, ranging from "excruciating" to simple expletives. Blurting out curses often brings knowing laughter from the group. The list includes examples they expect the listener has experienced or can imagine. "It feels like a toothache in my back." "It feels like somebody hit me with a baseball bat." Invariably, the group notices that some members don't contribute many (if any) words to the list, so we start talking about the numeric self-rating scales used today in clinical settings. I explain that the most common scale runs from 0 to 10, with 0 indicating no pain at all and 10 reflecting the worst pain you can imagine. Now the fun begins.

I stand up and, while gesturing enthusiastically with my hands and expressing cheerfulness with my face and eyes, tell the group I am having a terrible headache. "It started about 8 o'clock this morning over my right eye with pain boring into my head and flashes in my eye, then spread through my whole head so bad that I am sick to my stomach and I really should be home in a dark room taking pain medicine." Now I ask the group to put their hands behind their backs and on the count of three put their hands out in front, voting with their fingers on how severe my headache is on the 0–10 scale. "One, two, three, shoot!"

I have done this exercise with hundreds of groups over many years, and the results are always the same. Some people vote high, and some vote low. Often there are a 0 or two as well as 9s and 10s. Some votes are in the middle. So, one by one, I ask everyone why they voted the way they did, starting with the highest. It's not a perfect rule, but the patterns are amazingly consistent. People who have headaches themselves vote high for my headache, especially if my description sounds like their problem. The more my headache doesn't resemble theirs, though, the lower they vote, down into the 5–6 range or lower. For the most part, people who don't have headaches vote low, but the low voters have a very different line of thought. "You're here, aren't you?" They vote low because, to them, I don't look or act like I have a headache. People who vote in the mid-range usually are considering some combination of how I am behaving (observers) and what I am saying (listeners).

## COMMUNICATING PAIN

As the members of the group recount reactions of specific people to their stories of pain, they begin to understand a key principle in pain communication: the other person is half of the deal. This is particularly important to keep in mind in the doctor's office, as many patients with chronic pain report that physicians, especially surgeons, clearly are more observers than listeners and tend to minimize patient complaints. After all, the patients don't look like they have pain unless they are weeping, wincing, limping, or otherwise behaving demonstratively. They don't have a cast or stitches. They don't have objective consequences or markers of pain, such as fever or a fast heart rate. This is one reason why patients sometimes exaggerate their pain behaviors to impress the doctor with the severity of their problem, especially if they happen to be having a relatively good day in the context of many terrible days over previous weeks and months. Experts have devised physical examination signs to "catch" patients who are supposedly overreporting their symptoms or overacting. However, there are no blood tests or imaging techniques that measure pain severity in common clinical practice. More about this perfect storm of misunderstanding is coming in chapter 3.

> Roberta: "Before I got my back problem, I thought you had to be in a wheelchair or be like one of those people with crooked legs and those crutches that clip onto your arms. You know, like you could *see* that they couldn't do things like normal people. If I heard about somebody who wasn't working but they looked okay, I thought, 'lazy.' I know people around me think I'm weak or even faking my pain. Why wouldn't they? That's how I would have felt."

## GIVING UP

The final column of words in figure 1.1 reflects the frustration that frequently comes from repeated unsuccessful attempts to communicate chronic pain to significant others and to medical providers. Over time, people with chronic pain often try less and less to be heard and understood, leaving them with a profound sense of isolation and loneliness. Imagine not being able to share with people close to you your concerns about important life issues, such as money, work, or sex, and you will appreciate in some measure this loss of intimacy. This strategy of silence works well initially because it relieves the frustration of failing to get their pain across to another person. As time goes on, this silence severs the connection with loved ones, friends, and coworkers that is so critical to developing true empathy and getting appropriate support. For many people with chronic pain, this withdrawal leads to a dark inner sense of helplessness. After all, how can anyone expect to be helped when the other person clearly doesn't understand the problem? If you have ever had a problem that you cannot talk about to anyone and for which you cannot imagine a solution or even getting help, you know what is bound to follow: hopelessness.

Loneliness and the loss of hope are so common among people chronically disabled by pain that it is no wonder the vast majority are plagued by depression, fear, and anxiety. Whether these comorbidities precede the chief complaint of pain or result from it is often debated in individual clinical situations and in large-scale research projects, as if the solution to the primary condition will relieve the consequence. "If you weren't so depressed, your pain would go away." More than half of the participants in the FRP classes are taking antidepressant and/or anxiety-relieving medications. Conversely, the search for a pain fix is frequently charged by the idea that pain relief will brighten the mood. In desperation, patients often seek risky and unproven treatments, including multiple injections and surgeries, in hopes of relieving not only their pain but also their emotional suffering. Unsuccessful treatment is commonly followed by deep resentment and anger when the result fails to eradicate the cause of the unhappiness. This is especially true when the psychological situation is only minimally due to the pain in the first place. Postoperative visits with surgeons can turn tumultuous when the X-ray looks good, but the symptom relief is insufficient to alleviate the emotional mess. These visits are clinical nightmares, and they are common.

> Roberta: "One time my doctor tried to tell me my back hurt because I was depressed. She said there was this famous doctor who wrote a book saying people got their back pain from repressing things that happened to them in the past. Emotional things, like abuse and stuff. That really made me mad. If my childhood was my problem, how come I didn't have back pain before?"

At this point in the conversation, the patients almost always want to tell their own stories of disappointment and rage about encounters they have had with medical providers, focusing on the central problem of not being understood. I have to watch the clock and remind them that we have a lot more ground to cover. Besides, this is not a pain program. It's not really about pain, even though pain was what drove them to seek medical attention. It's about recovering the ability to have a good life, physically and emotionally, in spite of the inability to get rid of the pain.

## HOW MUCH SHOULD I DO?

So, I write on the board the critical question facing people with chronic pain every waking minute of every day: "How much should I do?" (see figure 1.2).

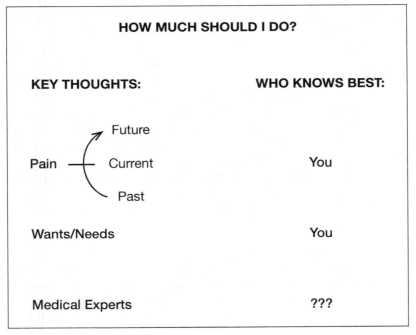

**Figure 1.2.**

This question comes in many forms and contexts. A person's train of thought can pass momentarily from "Should I go with my husband to the movies tonight?" to internal debates on whether to return to work or join the bowling league. Some questions seem simple and easily quantified: "Should I try to carry this bag of dog food into the house by myself right now?" Others challenge with complexity and timing: "I just had another injection and feel a little less leg pain. Should I try to start running competitively again or just try jogging alone or maybe with a friend? Should I try to make the varsity team this fall?" "What about sex? I don't know what to say to my new boyfriend." The FRP patients always struggle with this part of the conversation because they have too many function-related conundrums from their own experience to bring out. Rarely has any of them recently discussed these questions with any sense of being understood. So, the scene quickly becomes charged with the frustration of the moments of miscommunication they relate.

> Roberta: "They drove me crazy at work. My boss would watch me walk into the bank and see me chatting with my assistant in the hall and then call me in to tell me my time on the computer working up loans was not measuring up. You can't explain the pain of sitting too long to someone who doesn't have a back problem. They think you're lying or lazy. I tried to figure out how long I could stay at my desk and still be able to drive home and take care of the kids, but it wasn't that predictable. Sometimes I would close my door and lie on the floor. Once he came in without knocking, and that was really the end of me working there."

## GROUP COMPASSION

As the patients hear each other's stories, this can be the first time they realize that they are in the company of people who "get" what they are talking about and that they can talk about personally critical issues they have worried over but bottled up for months or years. Some of them visibly open up, reflecting their hope that this is a safe place to reveal their fears and failures. Others, who may not ever have felt comfortable discussing personal problems with relative strangers, remain withdrawn. The latter group used to worry me, and I would try to encourage them to join the conversation with tricky techniques I devised. I figured if someone was not raising his hand and talking, he couldn't be learning. He might be swimming alongside the boat but not getting on board. I gave up this practice of insisting on participation years ago. The group's wisdom grows over time and through organic pathways that I cannot drive the patients through. These people already carry with them most of what they need to know. They have just stopped hearing it somehow.

This is not my story to tell, nor is it my lesson to be taught. While there are basic truths and effective strategies to be revealed from their experiences, there is no one-size-fits-all formula to cram into these individuals. I have watched too many physicians try to force their version of the truth on very experienced patients, and I do not concede that this approach serves anyone. I have to trust the process of letting each person contribute and learn in his or her own way. In the FRP experience, people help each other primarily by just being their authentic selves in words and action. Also, these patients recognize foolery in each other with laser accuracy. It is the courage to reveal one's truth that allows the group to develop the understanding and knowledge that reflect to the individual ways of being and caring for him- or herself that are effective in the long term going forward into the real world.

While some patients are more forthcoming than others with their questions of how much they should do, everyone knows this is critical ground. Almost always, a certain discontent develops as the group runs out of examples and turns to me for the "answer" as if I am the one who should know how much they should or shouldn't do. This is an uncomfortable moment because the next layer of learning takes time, and I have to ask them to be patient. Occasionally, there is a groan. I must be holding out.

To get to the next layer, I ask the members of the group to pause for a moment and recall a specific time when they were trying to decide how much they should do. Then I ask, "What went through your mind? What were you thinking about?" The first response is always, "The pain!" Okay, so what about the pain? Here comes another example of a thought pattern common to people in chronic pain that is almost counterintuitive to their pain-free peers. The most important feature of their pain is usually not the pain they are currently experiencing. It is true that the present pain can simplify the answer when it is so severe that there is just no way the person can imagine performing the task in question. If you hurt so much that you can't get out of bed, sitting on the bleachers at your daughter's basketball game for an hour is not going to happen. As we will see momentarily, pain levels fluctuate chaotically for people with chronic problems, so most of the time, the current pain level is not the critical determinant in the calculus of activity decision making. "What's it going to cost me?" trumps immediate experience.

## PRIOR PAIN PREDICTS THE FUTURE, SORT OF

Paramount in every consideration of how much they should do is their prediction of how much pain the activity is likely to generate. And how do they know what pain the activity will produce? The group's unanimous response comes quickly. They have learned from past experience. So, I write "Pain: Future, Current, Past" on the board, as you can see in figure 1.2. Sometimes the prediction comes from recollection of exactly the same activity, an activity they may have performed many times over months and years. If the last few times you played on the floor with your toddler or sat through a movie you could hardly move for the next day or two, you are less likely to try those activities again. But it's not that simple. The association between a given activity and resulting pain is rarely hard and fast. If sometimes at the grocery store you have had to leave your shopping cart half full and hobble to your car empty handed but other times had no pain, today's decision to shop or not can be perplexing. Over months and years, people with chronic pain rack up gigantic catalogs of memories about activities and associated pain. These collections are massive and murky because the associations are complicated and confusing in ways that individuals really struggle to unravel and articulate.

So now the group is ready to dive a little deeper into the predicting-from-memory problem. Although we are going to discuss acute pain episodes another day, for now I ask them to recall a past episode of their own pain as clearly as they can. Then I ask them what they did to cause the pain. It's amazing to watch the members of the group react to each other's efforts to respond as they realize that clear cases of sudden-onset flare-ups directly following an activity or trauma that anyone might expect to cause back pain are relatively rare. "I felt a pop in my back as I was lifting a bucket of water out from under the sink." That sounds pretty straightforward to everyone at first. But it turns out that the pain didn't actually start until the next morning when the person tried to get out of bed. So how did the bucket of water cause the pain?

There are medical paradigms purported to explain such delayed pain onset. One doctor may explain the pain as a matter of delayed-onset muscle soreness, well known to athletes and weekend warriors. Another doctor may claim that the same delay is due to overnight mounting of inflammation in a torn disc wall. These "educated guesses" generally cause more confusion than clarity or reassurance.

In reviewing their own experiences with flare-ups of pain, most FRP groups admit that these narratives of strain-induced pain actually developed and became truth because the "bucket" was the only recent activity they could recall that was uncustomary and plausibly traumatic. And how about all the other things the person did in the days prior that were more taxing to the back than the bucket of water? What about the idea of "sleeping wrong" and waking in pain? The stories roll out. A new appreciation of the prediction challenge often comes with resistance at first, but the more the members listen to each other, the more profoundly the group recognizes that blaming specific physical activities for pain can be a very tricky business.

## FEAR RULES

What is not confusing or debatable for the group is the fundamental conclusion from all these experiences and associations with pain: fear of pain is the critical motivator in deciding whether to take on an activity. People try to be reasonable when applying their past experiences to their predictions, but fear of possible pain far outweighs recollection and logic. After months and years of such forecasting, a certain second sense of what to do and what to avoid mushrooms in the mind and compels people to make activity decisions that may not make any sense to the people around them.

Here is yet another element in the crucible of miscommunication. As difficult as it may be for a person to admit to himself that he is afraid to return to work or take his children on a canoe trip, it is much harder for him to convey this feeling to his boss or his kids. Being afraid is not easy to talk about, especially if you cannot substantiate your fear. How have the group members dealt with this taboo against expressing their fear as the true basis of their avoiding activities? "I can't do it because I have a bad back. I have bulging discs. My doctor says I have the spine of a 90-year-old. Besides, I tried it before, and I paid for it big time." Over time, these "reasons" can begin to sound like excuses and often become irritating to family and peers who are losing out in some way when unspoken fear of pain restricts or eliminates what would have been a shared activity. If you happen to be having a relatively comfortable day and don't appear to be in much pain, the fear is all the less evident or explicable, and the aggravation is all the worse.

> Roberta: "Really my boss wasn't that bad a guy. And the weird thing was that some days I could power through the day at my desk and my back would be pretty good. There were a couple of afternoons, though, when I couldn't get out of my chair, I hurt so bad. I had to wait 'til everybody went home and crawl out to the front door. I called a neighbor to come give me a ride home. It got so that I would leave work as soon as my back started acting up, so I wouldn't end up like that. I couldn't explain that to anybody, so I would just sneak out and go home."

Not everyone in the group is comfortable with this revelation of fear behind their activity decisions, but no one says it's untrue. The discussion often bogs down as this topic matures, so I try to refocus by asking what they would do if someone called right now and asked if they would like to go see a movie tonight. "What's the movie?" is about as frequent a response as "I hurt too much." Herein lies the great internal debate for people with chronic pain facing activity decisions. Asking about the movie reflects the person's need to value the activity. If the movie doesn't appeal to the person or the person just doesn't enjoy going to movies in general, the decision not to go is simple and has nothing to do with the person's pain experience or fear of future pain. You just don't want to go. What about waking up and remembering there is no food in the house for breakfast? Will you go to the market? Maybe breakfast is not part of your routine. Maybe the kids will wake up soon and they will be hungry. Maybe your spouse could go. How about deciding whether to go back to work next week? Maybe you have plenty of money and can afford to stay at home. Maybe you are already 2 months behind on the rent. Maybe your team at work needs your skills to complete a critical mission. Independent of your pain, desire and necessity drive these decisions. So, I add them to the board by writing "Wants/Needs," as seen in figure 1.2.

## WHAT MATTERS TO *YOU?*

There are many ways in which members of the group talk about what they value in their lives, but two features stand out. First, what they want and need varies widely between individuals. One member may be dead set on returning to active military duty, while the others cannot imagine such a future for themselves. Two members may both be considering returning to similar customer service jobs, but one is on workers' compensation and nearing retirement while the other has years to go and no other prospects that pay as well. Second, beyond the most basic needs for survival, people prioritize their wants and needs so differently. One person in the group may be driven to resume daily gym workouts prescribed by his cardiologist to prevent another heart attack yet fears returning to police work, where he may endanger his partner if suddenly incapacitated by an attack of back pain. In the next chapter, you will see how striking and complicated these differences can be between individuals.

> Roberta: "Honestly, I hated my job at the bank. The people there were all into themselves, and even office parties were strange because nobody really cared about your life outside of work. Customers would get mad at me for turning down their loan applications. That was no fun, for sure! But I had worked there so long, and I didn't know any other job I could do and make that much money. I was scared, and I needed the money to keep my home and get clothes and everything for my kids. I *had* to work, so I kept trying."

## THE DOCTOR KNOWS BEST. REALLY?

At this point, I remind the group that our current concern is the question, "How much should I do?" I ask the group perhaps the most embarrassing question: for me. Why not ask your doctor how much you should do? This question invariably generates a combination of howls and murmurs, as I write "Medical Experts" on the board. Their stories about physicians giving opinions on returning to work, sport, recreation, sex, and activities of daily living often range from absurd to tragic. Two people in one group had similar disc operations a year ago. One was told never to lift more than ten pounds, and the other was advised to return to any desired activity once their surgical wound healed up. They looked at each other in disbelief. How could they get such different answers to the same question? Who can blame them for raging over the consequences that these different opinions have had on their lives? Having listened to these stories for many years and asked many physicians how they feel about telling patients with chronic back pain how active to be, two things are clear to me. First, physicians are very uncomfortable making decisions when they have inadequate information, time, and scientific foundation. The brief clinical visit and exam room setting in which these decisions are usually made provide all three shortcomings.

The second conclusion is more subtle yet fundamental to the frequent failure of physician and chronic pain patient to connect effectively. Pain and fear are subjective and cannot be measured, so there is no way to plug them into an objective formula whose solution answers the questions of return to activity scientifically. This is why clear communication about the patient's personal history of pain is so key. Physician and patient must trust each other quickly in order to concur that the subjective foundation for their decisions is true. This trust is often severely challenged early in clinical encounters, as we will see in detail in chapter 3. It has been famously said that it is more important for the physician to know the patient with the disease than to know the disease in the patient. This is what they are talking about.

## WHO KNOWS YOU BEST?

So far, we have established that the key elements people consider in deciding how active to be are their personal memories and predictions of pain and whether they want or need to do the activity in question. Less important most of the time is the current level of pain, and physician input usually proves less than constructive. The next two questions are critical and always produce the same resounding and unanimous response. "Who is the world expert on your history of pain and in your ability to predict what an activity might cost you?" "I am." "And who is the world expert on what you value in life: what you need, want, and care about?" "I am." So, I add "You" and "You" to the board, as you see in figure 1.2.

Since physician input is generally feeble, the decision of whether to take on an activity rests essentially on the person facing the decision. This clang of truth brings dropping of tense shoulders and nods of assent: visible bodily reflections of the relief that comes from revealing and sharing a fundamental understanding that has long been obscured, even from oneself. The group descends into a quiet moment that evolves into a communal uneasiness with a tinge of despair. They realize that from one perspective, they are lost. No one can help because no one understands their pain. "We are so screwed." "So, now what?" "Thanks for pointing out how trapped we are." The revelation that each of them has the best information for deciding what to do in the physical world inevitably brings out frustration and anger but never disagreement.

## IT'S *YOUR* BACK AND *YOUR* LIFE

This used to be a scary moment for me. In early days, I would try to relieve the group tension or somehow change the conversational channel by telling a story or a joke. But in the times I kept my feet in the fire and kept listening to many groups reach this emotional moment of understanding, I eventually heard the next step in turning their lives around. There is another way of looking at the fact that they alone have the best information. They now realize that they can take back control of their decisions if they are willing to take on the responsibility to do so. They have a choice. This shouldn't be news to anyone. After all, they have known everything we have been talking about all along. If they have always had the best information, how did they end up in such miserable situations of pain and disability? They learned how all by themselves, and here is how.

I say "all by themselves" because the method by which people who are disabled by chronic pain got that way is usually invisible and frequently incomprehensible to people around them. As discussed before, virtually everyone else has experienced acute pain that resolved in a progressively downward curve to comfort and functional recovery. Only the minority who continue to have pain beyond the several weeks of customary healing understand the next feature of their experience. They

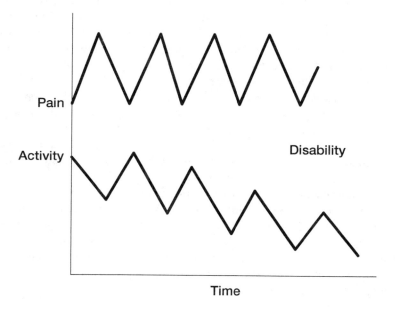

**Figure 1.3.**

don't have the same pain all day, every day, from day to day, or even month to month. Members of the FRP groups consistently report that chronic pain fluctuates up and down. There may be specific events that appear to exacerbate their pain, but they recall that, most of the time, the association of physical stresses and pain is vague. Figure 1.3, taken from the board, illustrates the learning curve of pain and disability. Actually, the curve is more like two diverging roller coasters.

## PATHWAYS TO DISABILITY

"When, for whatever reason, the pain goes up, what happens to your activity level?" "It goes down" is the resounding response. "Why?" "Duh, Doctor: because it hurts. I don't want to make it hurt more, and sometimes I just can't do anything." While there are many variations on this theme, the group strongly concurs that a rise in pain brings a fall in activity. "What happens to your activity level when you start to feel better?" "It goes up!" "Why?" The world does not stop turning when you have a flare-up of pain. The dog has to be walked, the paycheck has to be earned, the kids' lunches have to be made, your softball team needs you, and on and on. As the pain recedes, your list of things you have to do or want to do looms, and you choose which ones to take on and when based on your personal set of values and sense of urgency, stacking them up against your predictions of what each activity will cost you in pain. Over time, you have to make hundreds, even thousands, of these decisions. In doing so, you learn what things to take on and which ones to avoid. It's a messy process, often filled with more painful wrong guesses than pain-free attempts.

Sometimes the activity choices are obvious to an outside observer. Resuming your beverage delivery route, hiking up a familiar mountain, attending a wedding, and watching a sports event are examples of activities a person can clearly imagine and decide to pursue or not. However, the more subtle challenges have a more profound effect on the person's ability to maintain the basic facets of physical performance: flexibility, strength, and endurance.

## USE IT OR LOSE IT

I walk over to the door and ask who in the group has had a shoulder problem. There is almost always at least one person who has. I turn my left arm outward to grasp the door handle, turn it, pull the door open, and walk out of the room. When I return, I ask the shoulder veteran how I would do that if I had a painful left shoulder. "Use your right hand." "And what if I had a cup of coffee in my right hand?" "Move your feet so you can keep your left hand close to your body and open the door that way." Why are these responses so predictable and uniform? People with rotator cuff lesions or shoulder arthritis, the most common causes of shoulder pain, do not like to turn their forearm and hand away from their bellies (external rotation and abduction in medical terms).

Depending on their experience with musculoskeletal trauma, the group members vary somewhat in their knowledge of what happens to a shoulder or any other joint and its supporting muscles, tendons, and ligaments if you don't use them through their full range of motion and stretch and stress them. However, most members of the group have either broken a long bone or had a bad sprain or a joint operation that required several weeks of casting or bracing of an arm or leg. Why take the cast off at 6 weeks or so? Healing of the original fracture, sprain, or surgical wound sufficient to allow activity resumption is the key reason, but there is an equally important imperative. "What does your arm or leg look like when you take the cast off after several weeks?" Descriptors include "smaller," "shriveled," "atrophied," and "pale." "What does it feel like?" The limb is weak and stiff because muscles begin to shrink and weaken and connective tissues supporting joints start to lose flexibility and tensile strength almost immediately with immobilization. Even with good rehabilitation, recovery of flexibility, strength, and endurance can take more than double the time of restricted use.

These changes are obvious in the arms and legs simply by comparison to the opposite limb. You have only one spine, though, so the same anatomic responses to restricted motion and strain easily seen in the extremities are invisible in the back. Here is another reason people disabled by chronic spinal pain can be so misunderstood. They don't have a cast or stitches, bandages, or scars, and you can't see their spinal muscles. They don't look like they have a real problem like a broken bone. So, how could they be so disabled?

> Roberta: "People I used to see at the gym always told me how lucky I was to be slim. Recently, I saw one of them in a store, and she asked me why I wasn't going to the gym any more. She thought I must be doing some other workout, I still looked so good. I thanked her for the complement, but I lied and said I was roller-skating. I couldn't believe I said that. It was so stupid, but it was better than telling her I had back pain and lost my job so I couldn't afford the gym anyway."

Figure 1.3 shows the typical march to disability taken by people who make decisions to avoid activities that they have learned, rightly or not, could cause trouble. All is well if the pain just goes away. However, for those unfortunates who suffer through peaks and valleys of pain over months and years, this pathway of pain and activity avoidance leads to a physical and psychological inability to perform work, recreation, and activities of daily living. Even if you could find and fix the original source of the pain, you might not be able to reverse this deeply ingrained cascade of anatomic, physiologic, and psychological consequences. The end of this path is disability defined: the inability to perform activities critical to a good life. What that quality of life looks like we will discuss in chapter 7, but we need to work through more pressing concerns about the group's pain experiences before we can even approach that topic.

## WRAPPING UP

At this point, the group is usually exhausted. This has been an emotional hour of putting their personal cards on the table and discussing problems and challenges they have long submerged. Some wounds have been reopened. Some individuals feel reassured, even vindicated, by sharing such personal stories with others who seem to know what they are talking about without being judgmental or disparaging. They report varying levels of frustration at not getting to any solutions so far. They want to know how all this talk can lead to any real change, and they are still hurting. In fact, throughout the hour, pain has driven some members to squirm, lean on the table, stand and stretch, and even lie on the floor. I have not responded to their apparent suffering, leaving the group to wonder if I just don't care. The practice of not acknowledging pain behaviors constantly challenges me and the caregiving team. More about this comes in the next chapter on goal setting and training techniques.

To set the stage for the next discussion, the group and I review what we have learned from each other and settled on as common ground so far:

- No one knows your pain the way that you do.
- No one understands how you deal with your pain and fear in deciding what to do and how much.
- Disability evolves from this very personal decision-making process and its physical and mental consequences.
- You are the world's expert on how much you should do because only you know your history of pain and what really matters to you in life.

• *2* •

# You Can't Get What You Want
# 'til You Know What You Want

## STUCK

*S*ick and tired of their back pain, after months and even years of searching for relief, people often give up hope. Tangled up in conflicting and ineffective medical advice, fear of future pain, and quandaries about work and survival, it's no wonder they are confused, angry, sad, and sleepless. They feel stuck. They don't know how to get out of the mess they are in. They don't know whom to turn to. They feel helpless and hopeless.

Sound familiar? If not, before we begin today's class, take a moment to connect with these people's feelings. Perhaps you can empathize with one of the following scenarios.

Let's say you are sitting at your kitchen table. You stare at the pile of bills in front of you and realize that your credit cards are maxed out. You just cannot imagine how you can cut your spending to get even close to your income. You are smothering in a pit of debt. You have no savings and no plan. It's just going to get worse. You are stuck.

What if it's been 6 months since your spouse deserted you and the kids, leaving you without any explanation or support for your survival as a single parent? Even if you did have the skills, you can't get a job and an income in time to make your mortgage and car payments. You are way behind on your gas, electric, and phone bills. You don't know what to say to the kids, and you are too humiliated to talk with anyone, much less ask for help. Hopeless, helpless, and alone, you are stuck.

Hooked on alcohol? Are your worries and that uneasy stomach mounting through the day until you can get to that first drink in the evening and then several more to get to sleep? Every morning, you look in the mirror and see that heaviness in your eyes. You curse yourself for failing again, yet you are already taking mental inventory of your liquor cabinet and planning your next trip to the store. You've tried to quit or at least cut down a hundred times. You feel like crap, but you can't stop. No one knows you and your numbness because you just can't talk about it. You are stuck.

## EDDIE

Meet cherubic, 22-year-old Eddie, the tree guy. At 6 feet 4 inches, he looms over you, but his big smile and peach-fuzzed, rosy cheeks assure you that he is just a lovable bear. Three years ago, he suffered spinal and rib fractures when a coworker dropped a heavy limb on him from high above. He survived a long and painful hospitalization, but he became addicted to Oxycontin. He turned to heroin when his primary care provider tapered the Oxycontin. He tried to get off the opioids by reverting to his preinjury dependencies on alcohol and marijuana. His long-standing attention deficit disorder and anxiety seemed better, but not his pain. He couldn't walk across the street without a cane. His attorney pursued a personal injury case against his coworker for a large cash payout in lieu of a vocational training program. Tree work seemed an impossible dream, but it was the only way he knew how to make enough money to keep his home. Stuck and going stir-crazy at home, Eddie decided he had to get back on his feet somehow.

## WHAT DO YOU BELIEVE ABOUT PAIN?

Today's class is about getting unstuck. We are going to begin with what you and your classmates believe about pain and physical activity. Look at the "Beliefs and Goals" questions in figure 2.1. On a separate piece of paper, write down your own answers and any thoughts that come to mind. Tell yourself why you answered each question the way you did. Take your time. Most people entering functional restoration programs (FRPs) with chronic pain take at least 30 minutes.

# BELIEFS AND GOALS

1. Check one box to show how much you agree or disagree.

    a. The more pain people have, the less they are able to do.

        AGREE                                           DISAGREE

    b. People have to decrease their pain before they can increase physical activity.

        AGREE                                           DISAGREE

    c. I can increase my physical activities, even if I cannot get rid of my pain.

        AGREE                                           DISAGREE

*Picture the way you would like to be **4 months from now**. What truly matters to you? Take your time, then asnwer the questions below accordingly.*

2. Check one box to show how much pain is your goal.

    NO PAIN                                     MOST PAIN POSSIBLE

3. Beside each activity below, write what you really want to be able to do.

    WORK

    FUN/RECREATION

    DAILY ACTIVITIES

4. Your answer to #2 is your pain goal. Your answers to #3 are your activity goals. Check one box below to show which is more important to you.

    PAIN GOAL                                    ACTIVITY GOALS

**Figure 2.1.**

Now guess how hundreds of these people have answered these questions over the years. If you think they have all figured out the single, right "solution" to each item, you are dead wrong. They have answered in every possible combination and permutation you can imagine. Almost never do the members of any given group agree on any of the questions. They sometimes feel vindicated by what they are hearing from each other. Other times, they find their classmates' statements perplexing, even shocking. Eventually, everyone realizes that the greatest breakthroughs in understanding themselves come from listening to the thoughts and explanations of their peers. "That's crazy!" can reflect as profound a personal revelation as "I never thought of it that way."

Consider some examples. Look at your response to statement 1a: "The more pain people have, the less they are able to do." If you are in the vast majority of people who have not experienced chronic pain for themselves, including health care providers, you very likely checked "Agree." That is because most people's personal experiences with pain typically involve injuries followed by rapid recovery. If you have just sprained your ankle, the farther you walk, the more it hurts. What happens when you bruise your big thigh muscle and you try going down stairs? More stairs, more pain. Simple, right? Common sense! Besides, aren't you supposed to rest an injured arm or leg? Remember "RICE," the medical recipe for sprains: rest, ice, compression, and elevation? So how can it be that people who have had their pain problem for many months vary so much in their calculus of pain and activity? What are they thinking?

People who personally know all about chronic pain and agree with the statement that "the more pain people have, the less they can do" most frequently argue that when their pain is at a peak, they just plain can't do things. Sometimes, they can't get even out of bed. Considering "10 out of 10" pain, the answer is a slam dunk. For these people, it's black-and-white thinking. People who frequently experience a gradual crescendo of pain through the day report that they run out of pain tolerance and then just can't do any more. These folks disagree with statement 1a in the morning but agree with it in the afternoon!

> Eddie: "I couldn't help thinking about the stuff I used to be able to do. I used to feed trees into the chipper all day, then go bowling with my buddies at night, no problem. So I agreed with your first question, 'cause I figured most other people who aren't as strong as me would wimp out of what I used to do if they were in pain."

The physical demands of a given task further crystallize agreement with this pain-versus-activity statement. If you are considering bringing in a cord of firewood or climbing a mountain, even a relatively moderate pain level will hold you back. This is especially true if you have a strong fear of reinjury. So, people tend to agree that more pain means less activity by jumping to the assumption that we are talking about times of severe pain and very demanding physical tasks.

This black-and-white thinking turns quickly to gray when people recall that they don't have their most severe pain all day, every day. Virtually everyone with chronic pain acknowledges that their pain fluctuates up and down from day to day, even hour to hour. The relationship between pain and physical capacity gets fuzzy when you consider those days when your pain was pretty bad but you were able to do heavy tasks and your pain actually got better. What the heck?

The roller coaster of pain severity over time particularly confounds responses to statement 1b: "People have to decrease their pain before they can increase their physical activity." Consider a list of your customary tasks with the easiest at the bottom and the most taxing at the top. Let's say that watching TV is at the bottom and that playing tennis is at the top. If you had the same pain day in and day out, you might pick a point on your task list and say you can never do anything more demanding than that. As logical as that may seem, people with chronic pain generally don't think or act that way because the premise that they have the same pain all the time is wrong. This is one of the hardest things for other people to understand when they assume the pain is consistent from day to day. If they see a person with chronic pain going to the gym one day but hear that person say he can't go back to work, they don't know what to think. You can bet their thoughts are more likely critical than compassionate.

> Eddie: "Some days my pain kicks up, and I need a cane to get around the grocery store. If I'm having a good day, I still take my cane with me. People look at me funny if I don't. I know they think I'm faking it. So I use the cane even if I don't need it."

People who agree with the pain-versus-activity statement in statement 1a generally agree with the idea that you have to decrease your pain before you can increase your physical activity. For them, pain is inversely related to activity, plain and simple. The more you hurt, the less you can do. The less you hurt, the more you can do. Again, this minority position among people with chronic pain is also held by people who are familiar only with acute pain following an injury, like a sprained ankle. No wonder people who don't live with chronic pain can't understand people who do!

## WHAT MATTERS TO *YOU* MATTERS

Why doesn't everyone see that more pain means less activity? Priorities and mood commonly overwhelm this apparent logic. For most people, the importance or value of a given task trumps their pain level. If you wake up one morning with your usual aching back and realize there is no food for your kids' breakfast, you are going to go to the market, even if you have to shovel last night's snow off your driveway to get the car on the road. If you are a plumber and dread working in tight spaces under sinks, you are going to keep working despite your pain in order to get that paycheck. As revealed in chapter 1, the battles between the value of a task and the person's prediction of the resulting pain rage in the minds of people with chronic pain when they ask themselves, "How much should I do?" The same struggle confuses their assessments of pain and activity.

> Eddie: "Maybe I'm crazy, but I have to get back to cutting trees. Where I live, it's the only way I know how to make the money I need. I dropped out of high school so I could help my dad keep his business in the family. Now he's too old, so it's up to me. I can't really read much, so I'm heading back to tree work if I can. I don't care if the pain kills me."

The second driver of people's decisions as to whether their pain must decrease before they can do more is their mood. When you are down and out, even low levels of pain are hard to take. You just don't have the energy to pull yourself together and get moving. Some days you get so depressed with the mess you are in that you say no to everything. You convince yourself that just about anything is going to make your pain worse. The weird thing is that sometimes getting physically active actually makes you feel better both mentally and physically. So you know you "should" get moving, but you just don't. Depressed moods not only reduce your tolerance for pain but also alter your interpretation of the pain. When you are feeling low, you subject yourself to thinking that your pain is never going to go away, so what could possibly be the point of trying to do anything? Depression has a powerful negative impact on your predictions of the pain you will suffer if you try to accomplish anything physical.

Anxiety can have even more dire consequences, especially when it takes the form of fear of reinjury. Any logic you might apply to your decisions about pain and activity dissolves when your worries take over. Both anxiety and depression can drive people to conclude that they must decrease their pain before they can increase their physical activity, even though they know that activity can improve their mood.

## WHAT *SHOULD* YOU BE THINKING?

By the time the class has finished talking about the first two statements in the "Beliefs and Goals" questionnaire, they invariably look at each other and conclude that there may not be any "right answers" here. They can see that individuals have widely different thoughts about pain and activity and that their underlying thoughts inspire very different reactions and behaviors. By now, someone in the group has usually asked me what the correct answers are. If so, I still ask them to wait until we have discussed the third statement, partly because I know they are going to be disappointed.

> Eddie: "I just can't believe how complicated this is. It feels like I'm the only one who thinks like I do. I do get it that there's a lot more to making up your mind to get moving than how much pain you are having right now. I'm just so frustrated with all this!"

I can see that Eddie is not the only one in the group who is getting worked up. So, I try to pull them back together to look at the third statement: "I can increase my physical activities, even if I cannot get rid of my pain." Some people immediately dismiss the statement as ridiculous, because they are never going to get rid of their pain. Others note that this statement is different from the first two. This one is personal.

It's no longer a generalization about what *people* think. It's about *me*. There is a lot more energy in the room, and it's not all positive. The discussion frequently becomes contentious. Sometimes there are arguments. Behind everyone's response lies that person's belief that more activity will or will not make their pain worse. People who believe there is still a chance that their pain will go away or be cured someday wrestle with their peers who are convinced they will be in pain for the rest of their lives. They have very different attitudes about taking on more activity. It's personal. Occasionally, they try to convince each other to change their thinking. Almost always, the group's mood deteriorates, and they are not happy with me for stirring up the trouble. They want me to step in and resolve the conflict with the correct answers. What *should* they be thinking?

## WHEN THE EXPERT HAS NO ANSWERS

I refocus the group on the basic question of whether they will be able to increase their physical activities. My admission that I don't have a clue brings groans of disappointment. How could that be true after I have seen hundreds of people try to get back on their feet? Haven't I learned anything? Yes, I have learned that I am lousy at predicting who will be able to do what, and so is everyone on the staff, no matter how many months or years of experience they have had. This a scary turn in the conversation because the group feels betrayed. How can they trust me if I can't give them a formula for reactivating and guarantee them that they will be safe? They want to hear that all the scientific studies and our experience with hundreds of people add up to a single program that makes everyone hurt less and do more. Otherwise, how am I any different from all the other providers and promoters of the myriad treatments they have already tried and failed with? They bring out slogans from prior treatments, like "no pain, no gain" and "if it hurts, don't do it." How am I going to part the seas of conflicting advice they have received along the way? These are fair demands and questions, but the group is still not ready for the answers.

It's time to turn to the next section of the questionnaire. You are first instructed to picture the way you would like to be 4 months from now, to consider what truly matters to you, and to take your time. With this future self-concept in mind, you are asked to check one box in a row to indicate how much pain is your goal on a scale from "no pain" to "most pain possible."

I have asked hundreds of people without chronic pain experience and health care providers at medical conventions what box they think people who do have chronic pain check. "No pain" is the unanimous guess, but it is wrong. People with chronic pain almost never choose "no pain."

> Eddie: "My pain is an 8 out of 10 right now, and I picked 4 out of 10 as my goal. I didn't pick zero pain, because I know that's just not going to happen. I wish I could be a zero, but I don't even hope for that anymore. At least 4 would be better than 8!"

## IS YOUR GOAL *REALISTIC*?

Why don't people with chronic pain set zero pain as their goal? They don't believe it's realistic. "Realistic" is the key word in everyone's mind when they are setting goals, so much so that the groups often refer to the "R word." "Realistic," "measurement," and "deadline" distinguish goals from wishes, dreams, and hopes. You can wish you were prettier. You can dream about being rich. You can hope you will win the lottery. If you want to accomplish a goal, you are going to have to state your objective clearly and set the date for success. It's one thing to say you wish you could run faster someday. It's a whole different ball game if you say you want to run a mile in 10 minutes by August 1. Goals require concrete, measurable end points so that you and everyone else can tell you have reached them. You have to take *action* to achieve a goal. True, you have to buy a ticket to win the lottery, but beyond that, you are taking a passive role. Achieving meaningful goals requires real engagement and work. That's in part what makes believing that your goals are realistic so critical.

Where does your assessment of a goal as realistic or not come from? For most people with chronic pain, their past experience determines what they believe. All too commonly, though, someone else has contributed here. Many have been told by their doctor to accept that their pain will be with them forever, dismissing them with the parting words "learn to live with it." Those are some of the most dreaded words that patients with chronic pain quote from their experience with doctors, especially when the doctor has no ideas or instructions for *how* to live with it. A spouse or boss can turn critical in telling you that your pain will never go away, implying that you should "buck up" or "get over it," as if you have some basic moral weakness or character flaw.

## HOW LONG WILL IT TAKE
## TO GET WHAT YOU WANT?

At this point in the discussion, the group always turns again to me for the answers. Is it realistic to expect that their pain will someday go away? Again, I disappoint them. I honestly don't know, and I don't believe anyone knows. Even if I did predict the date of their relief, would they trust me enough to just sit around and wait for it before trying to get their lives back together? Now that we are speaking of time, questions about the 4-month deadline come up. Over many years of discussing goals with individual patients with chronic pain, it has become very clear to me that 1 week is too short. No one who has had pain despite seeking a solution for months and years truly believes that their pain and/or physical capacities can substantially improve in 1 week. Conversely, a goal of pain relief in 4 years is more like a wish or a dream because it requires no immediate action, no commitment. Many years of moving the goals deadline sooner and later have brought the consensus that 4 months is enough time to make real, meaningful change but not so long that action can be delayed.

Even though no one really can predict pain outcomes for a given person very well, there is no question that whether that person believes his goals are realistic matters profoundly. Whenever I ask a group, "What's wrong with having an unrealistic goal?" they first tell me they don't want to fail. Setting a goal they don't believe they can achieve is dooming them to a very personal failure. It's one thing to fail at a goal someone else has set for you and quite another to lose at a pursuit you have carefully determined for yourself.

Eddie: "My physical therapist told me that with massages and stretches she could get my fascia to move better and my muscles would be more balanced. I'd have better posture. She is a really nice person, so I went to all my appointments. But better fascia and balanced muscles didn't ring my bell. I don't even know what that means. If I'm going to get back working in the woods, I know I have to get stronger, like when I went to the gym in high school so I could play football. Man, I loved football! So, I worked hard, and it payed off. I could lift 300 pounds! It sucks that I'll never be able to do that again."

## QUITTING

While fear of failure comes out first in the group discussions of goals, it is not the most profound factor in the long run. Recovering flexibility, strength, and endurance cannot be done passively. It requires work. You have to do the work yourself. If you have a chronic pain problem, that work likely won't be easy. If you are working toward goals you thought were unachievable in the first place, guess what. When the going gets tough, it's easy to quit. A not uncommon refrain in early goal-based rehabilitation programs was, "Enough of this, my pain isn't any better and I knew I couldn't do it anyway." It took a lot of these hard knocks for me, the staff, and the patients to learn that getting what you want is much more likely if you believe it is possible.

## WHO DO *YOU* WANT TO BE?

As the group members read out loud their answers to item 3 in the "Beliefs and Goals" questionnaire, they realize how deeply different they are from each other. They may be similar in their pain scores, their treatment histories, and even their degrees of deconditioning, but no two people are alike in their goals.

Eddie: "I saw Frank this morning could only lift 10 pounds. He said he never could bend over right since his disc acted up. Roberta was right next to him and said she also had a bad disc, and 10 pounds was the best she could do, too. So now Frank tells us he just wants to be able to get back to doing oral surgery, but Roberta says she needs to carry at least 70 pounds to get back to her gym program. I could just barely do 20 pounds, but I'm trying to get back to cutting trees. No way the same program is going to get us where we want to go!"

Once group members reveal their different goals to each other, they invariably reach the same conclusion and raise the same question. There is no generic answer as to how much is the "right" amount of physical activity for everyone. There is no one size fits all. So their question is, "How does each individual get from his or her limitations to achieving his or her physical goals for the life he or she wants?"

## HOW DID WE GET HERE?

A little history is in order here to help the group understand how the program they are entering came to be. In the early days of functional restoration programs (FRPs), objective measurement of pretreatment trunk flexibility, lifting strength, and endurance for walking or running served as the starting point for each individual patient. Initially, we included all sorts of other physical capacity measurements. Over the years, it turned out that the abilities to bend forward at the waist, to lift repeatedly from floor to waist, and to walk or run trumped all the other parameters. Besides, they were easy for everyone to compare to the physical demands of their goals.

## NORMAL WAS NOT ENOUGH

Next, the staff would look up what the "normal" capacities would be for that person's peers who did not suffer from back pain. For example, 30-year-old men without back problems might be able to lift, on average, 30 pounds. So, a 30-year-old male patient in the program would be given a goal of 30 pounds. The course of training would then be plotted from his starting performance level, say, 10 pounds, to the "normal" goal of 30 pounds. The amazing thing about these early programs was that most program graduates with chronic work disability due to back pain were able to achieve these normative goals. These early results were published in the best medical journals, and accolades came from around the world. The functional restoration teams of physicians and therapists were duly proud, but there was trouble ahead.

As we followed program graduates over the years, we realized that many people were not satisfied with their outcomes. We were shocked when we learned that correlations were very weak between the physical gains people had made and their degree of satisfaction. Even pain scores did not match up well with satisfaction. Subsequent interviews with people who had graduated from the programs 2 to 5 years prior revealed a simple truth we had overlooked. We were embarrassed by how misguided we had been in our pursuit of normality, as if normal physical capacity would make a disabled person "normal" again.

Let's say you are the 30-year-old man struggling with chronic back pain and you hope to achieve your "normal" goal of lifting 30 pounds. If your chief goal in life is to be a piano tuner, guess what your attitude will be toward rehabilitation staff who are "making you" lift 30 pounds. They can't feel your pain. Provider–patient relationships were frequently strained by this well-intentioned approach to normality. Two fundamentals of modern medicine came under trial here. The physician's vow to "do no harm" was always in the back of our minds when encouraging program participants to work through their pain toward greater flexibility, strength, and endurance. Fortunately, the very gradual incremental training, leading day by day from the individual's measured initial capacities to his or her norms, proved to be challenging but safe. The second fundamental urge, to make a diseased person normal, was much more difficult to dispel. Medical victories typically include return to some normal status, such as reducing the febrile patient's temperature to the normal 98.6 degrees Fahrenheit and straightening a deformed spine or displaced fracture into normal alignment. By this paradigm, bringing a person's pain-limited capacities up to normal made perfect sense.

But what if you want to be a piano mover? How does that 30-pound normal lifting capacity serve you? It doesn't. Your achievement may look good to a statistician lumping your results with others

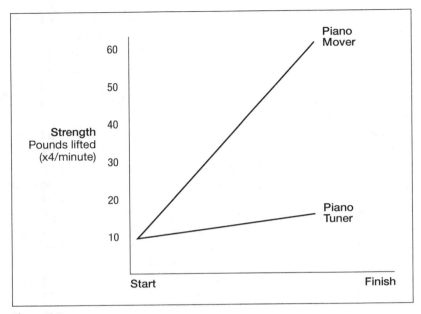

**Figure 2.2.**

who have successfully achieved their norms, but you personally will have failed. Whatever work you did, whatever pain you endured, will have been a complete waste.

## SAFETY FIRST

Figure 2.2 shows the training pathways for a piano tuner and a piano mover working toward their personal lifting goals. We have learned from thousands of people participating in FRPs over the years that this daily "small steps" progression from easy starts toward meaningful targets can work effectively and safely. This approach differs vastly from more traditional symptom-based training in which you do more when you feel good and you back down when you are hurting more. Taking advantage of those "good" days by suddenly increasing your training is much more likely to cause flare-ups than a steady course of gradually increasing your flexibility, strength, and endurance by small steps each day.

Take a moment to examine your own goals from the "Beliefs and Goals" questionnaire in figure 2.1. Return to the graph in figure 2.2 and on a separate piece of paper make a similar graph for yourself. Write in a "G" above the "Finish" point indicating the lifting requirement for your most demanding goal in figure 2.1. Next, write in an "S" above the "Start" point to show how much you think you can lift now. Draw a straight line from your start (S) to your finish (G), and you will see your personal program. Later in this chapter, you will find advice on how to accurately make training graphs for achieving your own goals for flexibility, strength, and endurance, but first let's have a look at your response to question 4 in figure 2.1, "Beliefs and Goals."

You have chosen the one box that reflects which is more important to you: your pain goal or your activity goals. You may have wondered what the right answer is to this question or at least how most people disabled by chronic pain have answered it over the years. They have checked every box on the scale, and virtually never do all the members of a given group have the same answer. This is yet another way in which people with chronic pain differ. When they reveal to each other the reasons and thinking behind their answers, they generally reconsider their responses to the statements in question 1. What you believe about the relationship between pain and physical activity profoundly drives your answer to question 4.

## WHAT MATTERS TO YOU MATTERS TO YOU

The most important takeaway from question 4 is the impact your response will have on your behavior. Will you keep trying to find a practitioner who might relieve your pain, be it through massage, manipulation, shots, pills, or (more) surgery? Will you give up on the medical profession and try to build up your physical capacities on your own? Chances are that if you checked the pain goal box, you won't find satisfaction in a gym. Conversely, pain pills or another injection don't stand much of a chance to help you achieve your activity goals.

Remember how frustrated the group was when I refused to give them the "right" answers to their questions about correct thoughts, outcome predictions, and realistic goals? Now that they have found the answers for themselves, I am going to play them back to you. First, if you are disabled by chronic pain, the pursuit of normalcy is folly when it comes to getting back your physical capacities for the activities that really matter to you. That is because only you know the thoughts and beliefs about your pain that guide your decisions about how active to be. The same is true for what you believe you are and are not capable of doing. Most important, only you know what is important to you in the major life categories of work, recreation, and daily activities.

> Eddie: "So you're saying it's up to me to choose what I want to do with my life, and I get that. Then I'm supposed to do a little more work every day to get there. But how do I know where to start and what to do every day? After all, I've been trying my best to keep going, but I'm so far from what I want to be."

## HOW TO GET STARTED

It's time to lay out the basic steps in FRPs that have helped thousands of people disabled by back pain for more than 3 months achieve their goals in life. You must first visit your most trusted medical provider and determine together whether you have cancer, an infection, a serious disease, or a structural problem with your spine that requires surgery. You need to rule out any medical reason not to exercise, such as an unstable heart condition, high blood pressure, uncontrolled blood sugar, and so on. This first step is explained in chapter 3. Once you have achieved this "medical clearance" and you are confident with it, you are ready to climb the functional restoration ladder toward the life you want.

Your program begins with some considerable soul-searching. What do you want to be doing with your life 4 months from now? Look at your goals from the "Beliefs and Goals" questionnaire in figure 2.1. Take time to make sure each goal really matters to you. Here are two steps that can help you. First, imagine that you don't have any limitations from your back. Second, in that physically unlimited state, consider what work, recreation, and daily activities would truly make you happy. One way to test the value and importance of your choices is to imagine yourself 10 years from now. Look back from that perspective at the life you won by achieving your stated goals. Imagine you are recounting your success to another person. Are you satisfied with and even proud of what you have accomplished? If not, reconsider and revise your goals until you can imagine them bringing you true satisfaction. This is a good time to make a facsimile of the worksheet in appendix A for your own personal use. Write in your goals for work, fun/recreation, and daily activities.

Now remember that these are your *goals*, not wishes, hopes, or dreams. You need some confidence that you can achieve them, and you need objective, measurable physical capacity targets and a time line for success. You may be able to figure out these physical needs for yourself, but more likely, you will need help from a trusted physical or occupational therapist or trainer. Armed with your written goals and medical clearance, one or two visits should do the trick.

For each of your goals, determine what you will need in terms of the following:

- Flexibility: inches from your fingertips to the floor, standing and bending forward at the waist with straight knees
- Strength: pounds you can lift in a crate or on a barbell four times per minute from floor to waist (see page 39)
- Endurance: miles per hour and duration in minutes you can walk or run

Now have a look at figure 2.3. Consider for the moment that your work goal is to be an office manager requiring 3- to 10-minute walks 10 times a day and that your recreational goal is to get your heart rate up to 120 beats per minute on a treadmill every morning to help you lose weight. Clearly, your recreational target is more demanding than your work target. Happily, if you achieve your treadmill goal, you will be able to handle the manager goal with no problem. This is the primary reason for targeting your physical capacity outcome according to your physically most demanding goal: you automatically achieve all your other goals. As the person in this scenario, let's say you have elected a goal of walking 30 minutes at 15 minutes per mile as your target, and you have written in a "G" over the Day 21 position on your "Endurance" chart

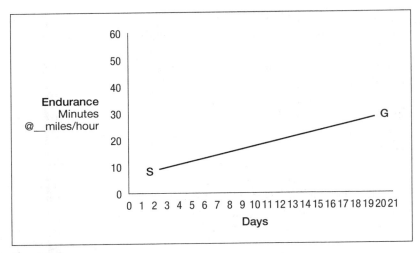

**Figure 2.3.**

as shown in figure 2.3. Let's say you are starting comfortably at only 1 minute of walking 15 minutes per mile, so you have marked your starting point on Day 1 accordingly with an "S." Draw a straight line from "S" to "G." That line will serve as your guide to how much you need to train every day to achieve your goal.

## CHARTING *YOUR* COURSE

Either alone or with your professional helper, write in the physical requirements of each of your goals in your personal version of the worksheet under the columns "Flexibility," "Strength," and "Endurance" in appendix A. Now it's time to complete your training chart in appendix B. Make out three graphs for yourself like the ones in figure 2.3, titled "Flexibility," "Strength," and "Endurance." Mark each of your graphs over the Day 1 and Day 21 positions to indicate your starting points and goals. Some goals will be harder than others to figure out how much flexibility, lifting strength, and endurance are required. You may find that your occupational requirements are specifically set out in a job descriptions or hiring manual. If you don't have guidelines for your work or other goals, you may need help from a professional skilled in this art. Generally, physical and especially occupational therapists are trained to do this. You have to make it clear to whomever you ask for help that you are looking for measurable targets for your goals according to your versions of the worksheet and training chart, both of which you should take with you to your appointment. The worksheet will reassure the therapist that you have been medically cleared by your health care provider for starting an exercise program.

You may also need help measuring your physical capacities at the start. On your own, you can bend forward at the waist, holding a tape measure and seeing how far it is from your fingertips to the floor. You can get a crate with comfortable handles and a set of bricks adding up to the weight you have targeted. (A standard red brick weighs about 5 pounds.) Get a timer and start your test by lifting the empty crate from the floor to your waist height four times in 1 minute. Add a brick and lift four times in 1 minute. Keep adding bricks one at a time, minute by minute, until you feel enough is enough for whatever reason. Use whatever lifting style feels right to you. Remember, you are trying to learn what you can do comfortably, not win a trophy. You can go to a track, walk around the block, or use a treadmill to get an idea how fast and for how long you can walk. Treadmills are best for most people because they display the speed and time for you. If you are going to a therapist for help, you can use their lifting and endurance equipment to test yourself.

## 21 DAYS?

You may be wondering where the 21-day time line came from. Observing thousands of people disabled by back pain participate in structured, gradually progressive training programs of varying durations has shown that most accomplished their goals (or as much of their goals as they ever could) in about 3 weeks. No one can predict how long it will take you to achieve your goals. No one can say with scientific certainty whether you will achieve them or to what degree.

## THIS IS NOT THE OLYMPICS

One thing is certain: this type of day-by-day incremental training has nothing to do with traditional physical training programs for athletes. In terms of gaining strength, athletes start training with capacities far above "normal" and aim to add perhaps an additional 10 percent, typically in 6 weeks or more. They are trying to build muscle size and strength. You are not going to build big muscles by doing the program in your training chart for 21 days. However, *on average*, people participating in FRPs over the years as much as triple their lifting capacity in 3 weeks. Something different from traditional weight training is going on here.

People disabled by chronic back pain typically have flexibility, strength, and endurance far below normal. They have reported in group after group participating in the FRPs that they got that way by learning not to bend and lift through the experiences and subsequent beliefs and attitudes we discussed in chapter 1. The solution that works best for most of these people for overcoming their deconditioning, stiffness, weakness, and lack of endurance involves gradual resumption of the very physical activities they have come to fear. By starting with easily tolerated levels of bending, lifting, and walking and building up step-by-step each day, most people are able to overcome their fears and beliefs and find themselves able to do things they care about.

> Eddie: "On a good day, my therapist would have me working on stretching and sit-ups and an exercise bike, stuff like that. But when my back was acting up, we would hold off, and she would use her ultrasound and hot packs and sometimes massage if it was really bad. I know she was doing her best, and so was I, but after 2 months, I couldn't really do any more than when I started."

## FLARE-UPS

This process of increasing exercise daily challenges everyone. Recall that chronic back pain rises and falls seemingly with a mind of its own. Of course, there are times when a flare-up is attributable to a specific incident, but not often. For many program participants, the most important lesson comes from realizing that flare-ups of pain almost always go back to baseline within a few hours or days despite hanging in there with the planned incremental training. This revelation, counterintuitive to many people thinking back on their responses to question 1 in the "Beliefs and Goals" questionnaire, can be the key to their recovery. A critical caveat comes when there is a new problem that needs to be professionally evaluated to ensure that there is no new injury to spinal nerve roots causing new pain, numbness, and weakness. True nerve root injury is extremely unusual in carefully graduated training regimens, and we will discuss how to handle assessment of injuries in chapter 6.

## START TO FINISH, IT'S *YOUR* JOURNEY

Before we begin the next chapter on going to see the doctor, let's recap the first steps you can take to getting your physical life back on track. Remember that this approach is designed to help people whose back pain has kept them from desired activities for at least 3 months despite best efforts to find relief from medical care. You will see that there is more to the story in the chapters to come, but here's how you can safely start your journey:

- Using your facsimile of the worksheet in appendix A, write in your 4-month goals for work, recreation, and activities of daily living. You don't have to have a goal in all three categories. Just make sure your goals are things you truly care about and believe are possible to achieve.
- Take your written goals to your next doctor visit and answer together the medical clearance questions on your worksheet. If you don't have cancer, an infection, a serious disease, or a structural spinal problem requiring surgery and you don't have a medical contraindication to exercise, proceed.
- Review your written goals and write in their physical requirements under the headings "Flexibility," "Strength," and "Endurance" with or without the help of a therapist or trainer. From these goals and physical requirements, make graphs like the

ones in the training chart in appendix B to indicate your flexibility, lifting, and endurance targets above Day 21.

- Test yourself or have your therapist test you to find your comfortable starting points for flexibility, lifting strength, and endurance. Enter these starting points in your 3 training chart graphs above Day 1 in your facsimile of appendix B.

- Connect the start and goal dots with straight lines in your three training chart graphs. They are your guides for how much bending, lifting, and walking or running you will do each day.

- On a calendar, write down when, where, and for how long you will train each of the 21 days you have selected. You can print out and fill in excellent calendars and daily schedules available online or in your computer's software packages. For many people, two sessions per day work best. Commit yourself to following your plan. Display your calendar where you will see it when you go to bed and when you wake up.

Now, about that doctor visit. Onward to chapter 3.

# · 3 ·

# The Medical Office Visit

"When you go to see the doctor about your back pain, what are you hoping to get out of the visit?" I have asked this question of hundreds of groups participating in functional restoration programs over more than 30 years. I have also asked scores of medical providers and researchers around the world how they think these patients respond to this question. The practitioners and scholars reply "relief" and "drugs." Year after year, the two replies that have come from the rehabilitation groups within 10 seconds are "relief" and "answers." Their responses are so predictable that I sometimes write down ahead of time these two words and "10 seconds" and put the note in my pocket. I then ask a visiting physician or medical student to write down the group's actual responses and the time elapsed. The visitors are routinely shocked to see that their notes and mine match exactly.

"Answers" means an anatomic and pathological diagnosis. "Which of the nuts and bolts in my back is my pain coming from, and what is the problem there?" These questions seem quite reasonable at first glance, so why are they so often overlooked or even avoided by the doctor? This difference in the expectations of practitioners and patients frequently opens a chasm of miscommunication that sooner or later sours the therapeutic relationship. Working together toward mutual goals requires a shared understanding and acknowledgment of the patient's demand for a diagnosis, especially if that demand cannot be met.

## FRANK

Meet Frank, the 62-year-old oral surgeon sitting next to you. He wears rimless glasses and a perfectly trimmed, salt-and-pepper goatee. He is nearing the end of his career operating on people with acutely painful lesions in their mouths. He has kept working despite a 10-year personal struggle with back pain, enduring long hours in the operating room with bracing and progressively higher doses of Vicodin. None of his professional training has prepared him for dealing with his chronic pain. He can't understand why the same short-acting opioids that have been so helpful to his patients don't work well for him. He can afford to quit working, but his vision of a physically active retirement of golf, skiing, and playing with his grandchildren seems a pipe dream. He can't even put his socks on without help from his wife! His pain has trapped him. He is not sleeping well, and he has to take naps between afternoon cases. His wife can see his depression and fear of the future coming on like a train.

## WHAT'S MY PROBLEM?

Today's functional restoration program (FRP) session begins by exposing a fundamental difference between people and cars. I ask the members of the group to imagine that their car suffers from an increasingly annoying rattle when they accelerate past 20 miles per hour. You take the car to the shop, fearing the worst. The mechanic comes out an hour later and announces that he is pretty sure the problem is somewhere in the front half of the car. Best guesses: 2 to 3 days and no more than $2,000, and your car will be back on the road. How do you feel about the plan, if you can even call that a plan? How do you feel about the mechanic and the shop, not to mention the whole world of automotive repair? Are you going to leave your car in that shop and shell out cash for a rental? Can you afford the time and cash to get a second opinion? How are you going to pick up the kids in time for school dismissal? Expletives would only fail to express your feelings, so you bury them in a sigh. If the guy can't give you a straight explanation of what nut, bolt, strut, or pipe is causing the rattle and what's wrong with it, how are you supposed to have any faith in the solution, if one is proposed?

Now consider this ugly afternoon with your car and think about taking your body to the doctor's office. Your back has been killing you for months, you've cut back your hours at work, your spouse doesn't understand you anywhere (but especially in bed), and you've canceled your vacation. The doctor looks over your questionnaire, asks you some questions, and then types your story into his computer. Next, he asks you to bend over at the waist, prods your back and buttocks, has you lie down and lift up your straight legs, pricks your legs and feet with a pin, taps your knee and ankle tendons, and has you stand and raise your toes and then your heels then try deep knee bends. His conclusion: "You have lumbago." Wow, finally you have an answer! So, now all you need is a definition of lumbago. It means you have pain in your lower back. But you knew that when you walked into the office! Okay, so the doctor seems like a really nice guy, and you don't doubt his sincerity. But how are you feeling about his "answer"?

The diagnostic verdict often proves pivotal in the office visit. If the doctor's explanation of your pain's source has not satisfied you, you may ask the doctor for tests. "Can we take a picture of my back?" You may be disappointed if the guidelines the doctor has in his computer do not call for imaging in your situation. You may already have had a magnetic resonance imaging (MRI) scan without identifying anything more than "age-related changes." You may insist on some test, any test, to try to get to the bottom of what is causing your pain.

> Frank: "One day in the OR [operating room] locker room an orthopedic surgeon friend of mine saw me putting on my back brace. I told him about my years of backache. He set me up to have an MRI right away. When I saw him in his office, he showed me the pictures and just said he didn't see anything to operate on. Pretty blunt, even for a surgeon. He offered to refer me to a pain specialist. I really felt lost, but I had to do something."

## YOU GOTTA BELIEVE!

The foremost driver of the diagnostic pursuit reported by people in the FRP rehabilitation groups over the years has been very consistent: "You can't fix a problem if you don't know what is causing it." Confidence in the diagnosis turns out to be critical to the patient's belief that the treatment will work. Hundreds of patients have told me about their moments in the doctor's office when they realize the doctor doesn't really know what is causing their pain. They basically stop listening. They don't even pay attention to the plan, if there is one. Doctors have often told me that they don't like taking care of people with chronic back pain because the patients don't follow through with their recommendations. They complain that their patients seem to either resist or just lose interest when they are prescribing the treatment, especially if the plan requires active participation by the patient. To be honest, why should either party expect compliance with a plan that is not based on a clear explanation of what is causing the problem in the first place?

On the other hand, you might be delighted to find a chiropractor who shows you your X-ray and declares that your spine is "out of alignment." He may have drawn intersecting lines with asymmetrical angle measurements to objectivize the crookedness you can see from across the room. Finally, a real answer. At least this is better than, "Not sure what's going on, but let's try a few weeks of me pulling your leg twice a week and see how you do." You are certain that this guy knows his stuff, and the plan to straighten out your spine makes perfect sense.

Next, you ask the doctor how long until you feel better. He says 6 weeks on average for your problem. That seems like a long time, but you can handle it now that you know what the real problem is. And you can't wait to tell your spouse and your boss, both dubious after all this time that your problem isn't all in your head, that your problem is *real*. A rock-solid diagnosis gives everyone credibility, especially you and the doctor. If you were originally injured at work and currently receive workers' compensation, you may finally be able to get your caseworker off your back about faking your inability to do your job. The diagnosis-based prognosis also makes her happy to know the case won't drag on forever so that her supervisor won't be chastising her for overspending on your case.

Paradoxically, the more dire the diagnosis, the more positive the credibility effect. If you tell someone your doctor says you just have a strain, that is not going to get you the sympathy you will receive if you have a fractured spine, spondylolisthesis, or osteomyelitis. Long, hard-to-pronounce Latin-based terms, like "sacroiliac osteoarthropathy," seem to carry the most weight, even if their medical merit is in doubt.

Almost everyone with unexplained back pain at some point worries that they may have a dread disease, namely, cancer, that has been overlooked. Often, they know or have heard about someone who went for months without a diagnosis only to finally find out they had cancer and then died. A diagnosis, even if it is wrong, at least rids the patient of this gnawing cancer phobia so common in our times and culture.

## THE DOCTOR BECOMES THE PATIENT

Once the group has brought out all these very good reasons to demand a diagnosis, I tell them I am going to be their patient. First, I am going to give them 10 minutes of what you learn about the anatomic sources of back pain in medical school. Then I am going to ask them to figure out what is causing my problem, drawing on their own experience. I want them to do unto me as they would have me do unto them. And they had better believe I want an "answer."

Medical problem solving rests heavily on the cornerstone of what is known as a differential diagnosis. So, I explain to the group how it works. The doctor listens to the patient's complaint and story. She then forms a mental list of the possible causes of the reported symptoms and winnows the list by asking pointed questions. Hopefully, the list is short and the doctor can move quickly to ruling out the wrong diagnoses and identifying one or two remaining possibilities. She then performs the physical examination for further clarification of the remaining suspects. Next, she orders tests to confirm the causative anatomy and biological process, such as a bone infection or a tendon rupture. Once the diagnosis is known, the treatment follows logically.

> Frank: "One great thing about my job is that I always know what I am dealing with. It may be bad news, like a tumor or a deformity, but at least the patient and I both know the score, the diagnosis. So the treatment makes sense. We're going to fix the problem."

Let's say you go to the doctor with a fever and a cough producing greenish sputum. The doctor asks you if you have any pain in your face, head, or chest; if there is any blood in your sputum; if you have recently traveled abroad; and if anyone at home or at work has had the same symptoms. The doctor is thinking of the possible anatomic sources: sinuses, airways connecting your nose and mouth to your lungs, and the lungs themselves. She is also thinking this is probably an infection, possibly viral or bacterial. She thinks tuberculosis is much less likely, not to mention the myriad other possible causes of cough. She takes your temperature, and you do have a fever. She listens to your chest with her stethoscope and hears crackles on the right. She suspects you have an infection in your lung, and an X-ray confirms you have pneumonia. She looks at your spit under a microscope and sees clumps of tiny blue bacteria and lots of inflammatory cells. Bingo! You have pneumococcal pneumonia. The treatment will be antibiotics, fluids, and rest, and you will be back on your feet in a week. You have your answer, and you are relieved. Thank God for doctors!

## SPINAL NUTS AND BOLTS

Ironically, the list of possible anatomic sources of pain in the lower back is short. Look at figure 3.1, and you will see the potential culprits: bones, facet joints, intervertebral discs, and nerve roots. I can't draw the remaining possibilities: muscles, tendons connecting the muscles to the bones, ligaments connecting the bones to each other across joints, and thin sheets called fascia running among these "parts," much like the

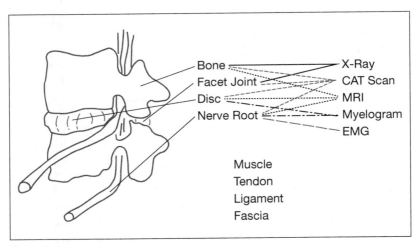

**Figure 3.1.**

silvery tissues you see covering pieces of meat at the butcher's counter. Let's consider the nuts and bolts one by one.

Anyone who has broken a bone knows that bones can hurt. The bones in your spine are called vertebrae, and they can break painfully. You have a pair of facet joints connecting the backs of the vertebrae at each of the five "intervertebral" levels in the lower spine. These facet joints are very much like the joints in the ends of your fingers, and we know they are pain sensitive because injecting them with strong salt water can cause pain in the back radiating down into the legs. The cushions between the vertebrae above and below them are called intervertebral discs. They are rather like very dense sponges contained by circumferential walls. The insides of the discs do not contain nerves, but the surrounding walls do, and tears in the walls can be painful. If some of the spongey goop inside the disc leaks out and pinches a nerve root, that can cause pain and numbness down into the leg along the route of that nerve. Everyone knows that muscle strains and bruises, torn tendons, and sprained ligaments can hurt because they are so common and so easy to identify and "diagnose" in your arms, legs, hands, and feet. Controversy clouds the fascia since some people believe it is the primary source of back pain, while others doubt it plays a role. The same can be said for the big sacroiliac joints that connect the lateral pelvic bones to the triangular sacral bone on which your spine sits, just below your belt line. None of this anatomy is news to the FRP group, as they are veterans of medical consultations in which these anatomic "parts" have been discussed, with or without images and drawings.

At this point, I ask the group how likely they think they are to discover which of the nuts and bolts in figure 3.1 is causing my pain by listening to my description and performing their physical examinations. "No chance" and "No way" are common retorts. "How are we supposed to know?" Fair enough, but I want answers. Often, some members of the group will suggest that my pain could be coming from one or more of the items on the list, citing explanations they have heard from their own doctors and therapists. When this does happen, the groups always realize that proof-positive identification of the anatomic cause of backache, through listening to the patient's complaints and examining their bodies, is rare. Even worse, this process is likely to provide different and often conflicting "guesses" from different practitioners. The shortcomings of the history and physical exam in nailing down a definitive and inarguable diagnosis are well known in medical publications, but these people have learned this frustrating truth through their own journeys from one practitioner to the next.

## IMAGING

I still want answers, so I ask the group what they are going to do next. "Get an MRI." I ask them what tests did *they* have first. The usual answer is an X-ray, followed by either a computerized X-ray called a computerized axial tomography (CAT) scan or another technique called MRI. A few people have had a myelogram, in which dye is squirted into the spinal canal and then imaged by either an X-ray or a CAT scan. Rarely today has anyone had a discogram, in which dye is forced through a long needle into the intervertebral discs to see if that reproduces the patient's pain, but discograms were popular for a while until it became clear that they were not very accurate. Some people with leg pain have had an electromyogram (EMG) looking for spinal nerve root dysfunction. As these tests are called out, I write each one down, as you can see in figure 3.1. I then draw a line from each test, connecting it to the anatomic parts they are capable of inspecting.

## SPINAL BLIND SPOTS

Most every group comes to two startling conclusions from this imaging exercise. First, even if you can see that something is not normal with one part or another, you cannot tell if that part is hurting. This turns out to be a critical flaw in the diagnostic process. I ask the group to guess how many out of 100 people who have never had back pain have a disc popping out into the canal where the nerve roots are (a so-called herniation) as shown by their MRI, CAT scan, or myelogram. They often know the correct answer is 20 to 30. They also know that "age-related" changes in facet joints and disc wear and tear are very common among people with no history of pain, and some have even had the experience of being told they have had a fracture without recalling any particular injury they can associate with it. They realize that most of the time, you cannot just look at a person's MRI and be sure that whatever abnormality you are seeing is actually causing that person's pain.

The FRP groups further realize that there are no imaging techniques that address the so-called soft tissues. These are the muscles, tendons, ligaments, and fascia that support the spine. They often recount their experiences with doctors and therapists telling them they have a problem with one or more bits of soft tissue because these tissues seem to be tender when prodded. Out of the hundreds of patients I have heard recall these diagnostic "moments," I cannot remember a single one that was substantiated by more than the simple explanation that "it hurts when it's poked." You have only to look at pictures of these tissues and see how small and intermingled they are to suspect the inaccuracies of tenderness on palpation. In order to push down hard enough to get even close to a facet joint, for example, you have to compress skin, fat, fascia, muscle, tendon, and ligament on the way. Further obfuscation occurs in the sensory strip in the outer layer of your brain, where you "feel" all the sensations coming in from all over your body.

Just to make diagnostic matters worse, all these soft tissues send pain and tenderness signals to the spinal cord and brain through the same little sensory nerves. Further, a given bit of soft tissue in your back sends pain signals to the brain through at least three different spinal nerve levels at the same time. No wonder tenderness is such a faulty locator of pain in your back.

## YOUR HAND VERSUS YOUR BACK

Look at your left hand for a moment, palm up. With your right hand, take a toothpick or a pin and very lightly poke the pad at the end of your finger. It's easy to tell exactly where and what you are poking, right? Your skin. Now bend the last joint in that finger sideways, with just enough force to create discomfort in the side of the joint. That pain is coming from the ligaments that support the joint. Nothing else responds painfully to that strain. Now pinch the big muscle just below where your thumb joins your palm. That deep ache is muscle pain, plain and simple.

It turns out that the chunk of sensory cells in your brain responsible for analyzing signals coming in from your hand is far more sophisticated and gigantic compared to the morsel that oversees your entire spine. This situation is key to your survival because you need to know exactly where things are happening in your hand to perform all the critical tasks your hand has to do, even when you are not looking. Not so with your back. The commonality of peripheral sensory nerves supplying all the soft tissues at each spinal level in your back and the relative deficits of the brain segment responsible for analyzing signals from those "parts" make it impossible for you to tell which part is generating your pain.

> Frank: "When the pain specialist pressed his fingers into my back and it hurt, he brought out my MRI and showed me how ratty my facet joints looked. My wife, Marge, was with me, and he noticed the joints in the ends of her fingers were knobby. He said that was osteoarthritis just like what was happening in my facet joints. He said injections should do the trick, so I said go for it. I did ask Marge on the way home, though, if her fingers ever hurt. It gave me pause when she said no."

## BACK TO MY CASE

So now I tell the group that I bent over last week and suddenly felt a pulling sensation in my lower back. I woke up the next morning with pain shooting down into the back of my left thigh to the knee. I am coming to them for help, and I want answers. Where is the pain coming from, and what is going on there? So, what are they going to do? Someone in the group almost always blurts out, "Get an MRI," but I plead for order in their thinking through my differential diagnosis. What would they like to ask me about my problem? "How bad is the pain?" "Does it hurt more when you bend over?" "Does it go away when you lie down?" "Is your foot numb?" "Are you controlling your bowel and bladder okay?" "Is your leg weak?" "What have you tried so far to get rid of the pain?" "Have you been sick in any way lately?" These are all questions they recall having been asked themselves. I respond that my leg hurts like hell, but I don't have numbness, weakness, or any trouble controlling my stool or urine, and I haven't been sick. I ask them what they think is wrong with me and where the problem is. "It's in your back" is about as close to a diagnosis as any group ever gets from the facts so far. They don't have a clue what the painful part and process may be.

Now we move on to the physical exam. They want to poke my back, but I tell them I'm not particularly tender unless they really push hard. Again, tenderness is a perplexing finding, especially when you realize that even normal tissues can be tender if you poke hard enough. They ask me to bend over at the waist, and that hurts, but it doesn't hurt when they ask me to lie on my back and they raise my painful leg. My sensation in my legs and feet is okay, and my calf and thigh muscles are strong. My ankle and knee reflexes are good.

## HOW DO THINGS LOOK UNDER THE HOOD/SKIN?

The group wants an MRI. I tell them my MRI report lists a short paragraph of abnormalities for each of the five levels in my lower spine. Degenerative disc disease, annular tears, facet joint arthropathy, synovial cysts, multiple bone spurs called osteophytes, hypertrophy of the ligamentum flavum, foraminal narrowing, spondylolysis of the pars interarticularis—on and on goes the list. The members of the groups have heard most of these terms before because they have popped up in their own imaging reports. Frequently, one of the members recounts getting a phone call from their primary care provider, who reads them their findings over the phone. Since it is a rare primary care doctor who can accurately interpret the MRI pictures for him- or herself, neither the caller nor the patient can appreciate what findings in the report are important and what ones are not. It is a rare patient who, on hearing all these medical terms, does not fear the worst.

There is a double whammy here. Radiologists, the doctors who officially interpret the MRI pictures and file the reports, are bound and determined not to miss anything that is not normal. So they report *everything* that looks abnormal. Remember that the point of the MRI is to confirm or rule out the presence of the single problem that the ordering doctor theoretically conjured up from the differential diagnosis. The radiologist usually does not know much about the patient, nor does she know the differential diagnosis beyond general labels on the order form, like "low back pain" or "sciatica." Therefore, the primary care doctor is stuck with a list of 20 or more abnormalities without a clue as to which one is the root cause of the patient's problem. So, how is the patient supposed to know what the problem is? All these medical terms sound pretty serious. At this point, both doctor and patient jump to the same conclusion: it's time to see a specialist.

Before we call the specialist, I ask the group to guess their chances of making a definitive, clear-cut diagnosis that multiple specialists would agree on when confronted by 100 patients with chronic back pain. To clarify the question, I ask them to imagine that they are going to see these 100 patients next week in the office. They get to ask all the questions they want, perform any physical examinations, and order any imaging they feel is indicated. All 100 patients return the next week wanting to hear what is actually causing their back pain. How many of the 100 does the group think they will be able to give the correct answer? There is usually a cynic in the room who shouts "zero." Most of the guesses range from 20 to 80. When I ask them to consider their own experiences, they are not surprised to hear that the true answer is less than 15 out of 100.

## WHO YOU SEE IS WHAT YOU GET

So, why have they each received several different diagnoses from the various practitioners they have consulted? Remember how desperately everyone wants an answer and for what reasons? Health care providers, especially those who specialize in back problems, recognize that desperation and often respond to it by making their best guess according to their training and the explanatory models they believe in. That is how the same patient may be told by an osteopath that he has sacroiliac joint dysfunction. His physical therapist says he has sticky fascia. His chiropractor says his spine is crooked. His acupuncturist says his chi is not flowing right through his meridians. His neurosurgeon tells him that at least there is nothing to operate on, but his orthopedic surgeon says his spine is unstable and needs a fusion. I have never heard an FRP group not acknowledge that this multiple-diagnosis conundrum happens whenever you consult more than one practitioner. They have lived through this confusion themselves.

When I remind the group that I am still waiting for an answer, you can feel the frustration building up in the room. So, I ask them to relax for a moment and imagine that their day of doctoring is coming to an end. Suddenly, 100 people call the office complaining of back pain that started earlier that day. There is no way to see all those people today, so you tell your receptionist to have all the callers just to do the best they can and call you back in 1 week. All 100 people call back in 1 week. Guess how many are all better? The group invariably splits up on this quiz. Someone usually says that no one is better, and most guess between 10 and 20.

## BACK ATTACK: MOST LIKELY OUTCOME?

Look at figure 3.2, and you will see their 1-week responses as X's. Now look at the X's showing their guesses for 3 weeks and 3 months later.

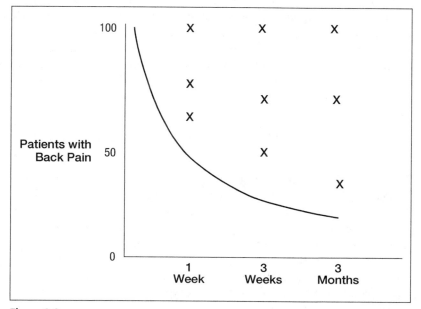

**Figure 3.2.**

Imagine now that you are one of the 100 callers on day 1. If you believe you have no chance of recovering without seeing the doctor in 3 weeks or even in 3 months, you are going to think and behave very differently compared to someone who believes he has a 90 percent chance of getting better no matter what. Right? So, it is critical to know the average natural history of an episode of sudden-onset back pain and whether it is a first-time experience or a flare-up of a chronic problem. This spontaneous recovery is represented by the curve in figure 3.2.

Remember that the room is full of people who did not recover and stay pain free as suggested by the curve on the time line. Their initial shock dissipates when they reconsider their own experiences with flare-ups of their own pain, and they recall that their pain almost always returns to baseline even faster than the recovery curve on the board. A note of caution is due here. Notice that the recovery curve does not fall to zero pain for all. In fact, back pain that lasts beyond the usual tissue healing period of 6 to 8 weeks required by such familiar injuries as fractures and sprains generally persists for months if not years. Patients in the FRPs commonly report that 3 months after their pain began, they suffered through the peaks and valleys of pain we discussed in chapter 1, but the pain just doesn't go away. All too often, they have progressively limited their activities to the degree that they have become so stiff and out of shape that they can no longer do the things that matter to them. They have become deconditioned and disabled, unlike most people who recover uneventfully from their episodes of back pain.

## YOUR CAR VERSUS YOUR BACK

Now they are ready to learn the difference between cars that rattle and people whose backs hurt. Rattles don't go away unless you fix them. Low back pain episodes usually get better without any particular treatment. That is why there are so many different treatments out there. They all appear to work, largely because most people go for treatment when they are in the middle of a pain attack or flare-up and are very likely to get better no matter what the treatment may be. That is how so many practitioners of so many different types stay in business. It is true that a diagnosis-based treatment can be successful. Think of the patient with leg pain from a herniated disc waking up pain free after having an operation to remove the disc fragment from the nerve root. Hooray, another victory for modern medicine. But the people in the FRP room have not had that experience, so now they want to know two things. They want to know how anyone can tell which treatments work and which ones don't. They also wonder why practitioners keep providing treatments if they don't really work.

## RANDOMIZED CONTROLLED TRIALS

It's time to explain randomized controlled trials (RCTs), the bedrock of evidence-based medicine. Let's say you want to find out which of two treatments is better for treating a certain disease. For example, you want to know if surgery is better than radiation for treating squamous cell cancer of the lung. You would start your trial by collecting lots of patients with this type of cancer who are willing to participate in your experiment. You have to be able to explain to them honestly that you don't know which treatment is better, and you have to tell them all the known risks of the therapies. You are not allowed to have a personal financial interest in the outcome. You must promise a board of human experimentation that you do not have any such conflict of interest. You must also be patient. It may take several years for you to write your grant proposal, receive funding after two tries, perform the RCT itself, and then collect and publish the results. If your results are impressive, it may take another decade for them to have an impact on clinical practice in the real world.

Forging ahead, you divide the patients with lung cancer into two treatment groups of equal size, assigning each person to one group or the other randomly through a computer program. If you really think neither surgery nor radiation will work, you might divide the initial patient sample into thirds and give the third group no treatment. One year later, you count up how many people in each group are dead and how many are alive, and you compare the outcomes of each group. You have to enlist enough patients so that you are sure you can detect a difference in outcomes if there is one. You have to be confident that the two groups are essentially identical in all features besides the cancer that could bias the outcome.

Let's say you start with 1,000 people and divide them into 500 for surgery and 500 for radiation. If 250 are alive in each group at year's end, there clearly is no difference. If 500 of the surgical group are alive and all of the people who got radiation are dead, surgery is the obvious winner. RCTs almost never come out so clearly. Usually, the outcomes have to be analyzed with statistical methods to determine the degree of certainty that whatever difference has been observed didn't just happen by chance.

## OKAY, SO WHAT *DOES* WORK FOR BACK PAIN?

Over the decades that RCTs have been applied to people with low back pain, there have been no home runs for any given treatment. One study may slightly favor one treatment over another, but the next shows no real difference or even the opposite result. Low back pain has been a particularly difficult nut to crack with RCTs. First, low back pain is just a symptom, not a discrete disease like lung cancer. Under the umbrella of low back pain lie many different causes, most of them unknown to the researchers and the subjects. Unlike the dead or alive binary outcomes for cancer, outcomes for low back pain come in the much fuzzier forms of scores from questionnaires attempting to measure pain and its functional consequences. As we have seen in previous chapters, these generic, expert-generated questionnaires are poor indicators of an individual's satisfaction with their outcomes, raising doubts about their validity. The assumption that the groups in low back pain RCTs are equal in all aspects is fundamentally flawed by the vast differences between individuals' goals and how they value pain and functional results. The group members know these person-to-person disparities only too well from listening to each other's goals and outcome preferences, as described in chapter 2.

> Frank: "The medical school's librarian helped me look up studies of radiofrequency ablation as a treatment for back pain. I have to say the articles I read were not that encouraging. I went ahead with the treatment, though. I just couldn't stand the idea of doing nothing."

## WHAT TO DO WHEN THE EVIDENCE IS IFFY

The lack of clear therapeutic champions for chronic back pain has led to two campaigns in the medical world. Clinical guidelines have been established by various professional groups to suggest treatments based on the best studies available. Overall, the guidelines are collections of possible treatments that could be tried, but there is no "one size fits all" for back pain. None of the guidelines recommends a specific, solitary treatment for chronic back pain. The second movement generated by the haze of treatment uncertainty has been shared medical decision making. This approach involves the doctor delivering to the patient the best available information and then giving the patient part or all of the power to decide what treatment to try. Neither of these two approaches has proven particularly effective. The group members who have had experience with one or both routinely complain that they were more confusing than helpful.

Now the FRP group wants to know why doctors and therapists keep prescribing and performing treatments that don't have a winning track record in RCTs. Remember that RCTs look at large groups of people, not individuals. In each treatment group, there are people who do well and people who do poorly, with most people in the middle, as in a bell-shaped curve. There is no way for a doctor to predict from the results of an RCT how her next patient is going to do. If you are that next patient, all the RCTs in the world don't help much if they haven't shown much difference between your treatment choices in the first place.

So, how do doctors decide which treatments to recommend to their patients? I ask the group if they have ever experienced lack of improvement after a treatment. All agree. Did you go back? No. Did you even cancel your follow-up? No. Did your practitioner call to see how you were doing? No. Did you ever have a treatment that helped? Yes, at least sort of. Did you attend your follow-up appointment? Yes, and I said how grateful I was. I even brought chocolates for the office staff. Okay, so if you were a doctor and your patients behaved like you have as a patient, following up if happy and disappearing if not, over time how would you feel about your treatment? It works! Right? Over time, this impression is hard to beat with RCTs, especially when you consider that most patients with acute back pain or a flare-up get better regardless of the treatment. "I know my treatment works because I've seen it over and over." That's why different practitioners keep treating with what they believe works, even if their treatment has not clearly prevailed in RCTs. They are all the more likely to persist with treatments they know will be reimbursed by insurance carriers.

## SAY, WHAT ABOUT INSURANCE CARRIERS?

The comparison of the for-profit health insurance industry to a casino has come up so many times over the years that I can't help wondering if there is some truth to it. I don't pretend to be an expert on health insurance; in fact, I can't even understand my own medical bills, but here is how the story goes. First, imagine that everyone is healthy all the time. No health insurance industry, right? No losing gamblers, no casino. You buy health insurance to protect yourself and your dependents or employees from the medical expenses of getting sick or injured. So how much should that protection cost? Just like casinos, the insurance companies are allowed profits as percentages of their margins between revenues and costs. Therefore, the sicker and more demanding of health care the insureds are predicted to be, the more premium dollars the insurance carriers can charge and take to the bank, even better to the stock market. The carriers make out well as long as they keep paying the expenses of treatments that they agreed to pay for when setting their premiums at contract time. The bigger the pie, the bigger the piece. If you were a carrier in this scenario, it would be fine to pay for treatments that don't work because you care about your profits, not health outcomes.

## PAYDAY

When the subject of payment for health care comes up, I ask the group if they ever had to pay for a treatment even if it didn't work. Of course, they did. This recollection brings another "aha" moment. In the fee-for-service system dominant in the United States, health care practitioners are paid for performing treatments regardless of their outcomes. Every group appreciates the potential impact on our health care economy should insurance reform demand proof of success before treatment is paid for. No one believes this will happen anytime soon.


## A SPINAL ODYSSEY


At this point in the session, stories of chasing the diagnosis and treatment dream roll out from the group. Here is a common scenario. Someone with back pain consults his primary care doctor, who says it's probably a strain and there may be inflammation. The treatment is a short course of oral steroids. Three weeks later, the person is no better, so the doctor sends him for physical therapy. The therapist says his core muscles are weak and recommends 6 weeks of exercises, cautioning him to back off on bad days. Still no better, our patient returns to the primary doctor, who consults the guidelines and suggests manipulation. Next, a chiropractor takes an X-ray and diagnoses segmental subluxation. After 6 weeks of manipulations twice a week, the X-rays look a little better, but the pain remains. Frustrated, the patient demands that his doctor send him to a *real* expert, a surgeon. After waiting 8 weeks for the appointment, in less than 5 minutes the patient is told that surgery probably won't help. The surgeon recommends that the patient consult a pain specialist, and his parting words are, "If your pain gets so bad you can't walk, come back, and I'll fuse your spine with screws and cages." Spooked by the prospect of a big operation, the patient waits another 6 weeks to see the pain specialist. After finding tenderness over the sacroiliac joint, the specialist pronounces that joint guilty of generating the pain all along. He has a few choice insults for the practitioners who missed this obvious diagnosis. An initial steroid injection into the joint doesn't work. So, the patient signs up for "burning the nerves" that supply the joint. Before the treatment, called radiofrequency ablation, the insurance carrier demands the patient undergo two sets of test injections, which require another 6 weeks to schedule and perform. The day for the radiofrequency ablation finally comes and goes with no relief.

Eight months after their first encounter, the patient returns to his primary doctor. The bills for all his treatment have been rolling in, so far more than $30,000. The doctor hardly recognizes the patient, who has put on 40 pounds and needs a shower. Adding anxiety, depression, and insomnia to the problem list, the doctor recommends counseling. "So you think this is all in my head?" "No, I just don't know what else to do."

This session on going to see the doctor always runs overtime. The group is always upset, but there is a sense of camaraderie that comes from sharing their stories of pursuing diagnoses and treatments in vain. I sympathize with them and reassure them that I have heard similar stories from hundreds of people who came here before them. I know they are telling the truth without exaggeration. I acknowledge their frustration and anger.

## SO, WHAT DO WE DO NOW, DOC?

Now they are ready to hear what I recommend for future medical encounters to people disabled by back pain for more than 3 months.

Visit a medical doctor you can trust. Take any imaging or reports you may have with you. Make out your own version of the worksheet in appendix A and take that with you, too. Read to the doctor the goals you have written down for work, recreation, and daily activities 4 months from now. Ask the doctor for *answers*—not for a diagnosis but for answers to the three questions below:

- Do I have cancer, an infection, a recent fracture, or any serious disease that can be treated effectively?
- Do I have a structural spinal problem that requires surgery?
- Do I have a medical reason not to exercise?

If all the answers to these questions are "no," you are ready to proceed with the program laid out in chapter 2 and in your training charts. This is also a good time for you and the doctor to review your experience with drugs. Chapter 4 tells you how and why.

# Drugs

$\mathscr{I}$ guarantee you: when I announce that we are going to talk about "drugs," the functional restoration program (FRP) group will react with a mixture of snickers and silent shock. They will be shocked because doctors just don't use the word "drugs" when speaking to patients. Medical providers properly use the word "medications." But "drugs" and "medications" refer to the same substances, so I'll ask the group, "What is the difference?"

We start with the members of the group who snickered. What were they thinking? The word "drugs" connotes to them something sinister, even illegal. Good citizens take medications, while criminals and degenerates do drugs. Remember the war on drugs? There has never been a war on medications. So, what personal experiences do they recall that brought such an immediate negative reaction? Their stories primarily involve two classes of sedating substances: opioids (oxys, percs, vikes) and benzodiazepines (benzos, chill pills, tranks). Marijuana sometimes makes the nefarious list as well.

## WESLEY

Meet Wesley. He is sitting down at the end of the table today, the burly and balding African American man in the gray T-shirt with "ARMY" in black letters across his chest. He is a 29-year-old sergeant. A year and a half ago, the armored vehicle he was driving in Iraq was blown up by a mine. Three of his squad were killed immediately. He woke up in a hospital in Germany with no recall of recent events. After 6 months in a rehabilitation facility in the United States, he continued to have back pain and numbness radiating into his right foot. No operable lesion was seen on magnetic resonance imaging. He got partial but only temporary help from three epidural steroid injections. Neurontin was not helpful and made him dizzy. His thinking and memory straightened out, but you have noticed he has an awkward gait, listing to the left as he walks down the hall. He feels deep remorse for his dead comrades, and he vows to return to his unit.

## OPIOIDS

In the 1980s, the FRP groups would on average include a few patients who had experience with what would now be considered low doses of opioids, such as oxycodone or codeine, usually compounded with acetaminophen, whose brand name is Tylenol. Once the most prescribed drug in the United States, physicians commonly ordered the benzodiazepine Valium for their anxious patients, and FRP participants frequently took this medicine for its purported ability to relax tense muscles. Some patients admitted to using marijuana but primarily for recreation and not to treat their pain per se. In those days, the group sessions did not run to discussions of the illegality of the opioids and sedatives because medical doctors were prescribing them and patients were taking them with what FRP participants considered to be positive attitudes. There was very little prescription drug–related criminal behavior, and accidental overdose was almost unheard of.

The opioid epidemic that has gripped the United States in the past 30 years profoundly altered the FRP group discussions of drugs. Through the years, more and more participants came into the programs taking higher and higher doses of opioids. Recently, a sea change of relevant media has progressed from medical praise for liberalizing opioid prescription for pain to recognition that the pendulum has swung too far toward criminality and death by overdose.

Over time, the FRP sessions on drugs deteriorated into arguments about the right way to deal with opioids. These were often contentious debates, ending inconclusively and breeding bad feelings and distrust that invaded the therapeutic relationship critical to good medical care. Early in my medical career, starting in 1981, two experiences had shaped my attitude against the trend toward more liberal opioid prescription. The first was being physically threatened in my office by a gigantic and belligerent patient when I questioned his demand that I refill oxycodone prescriptions initiated by a departed partner in my practice. The second came when an opioid-addicted patient burned to death after falling asleep smoking in bed. I became a medical maverick in my community inasmuch as I rarely prescribed opioids, virtually never for chronic pain. I also encouraged patients who were taking opioids long term to quit if they wanted to enroll in the FRP. Many patients who did so were surprised to experience higher levels of energy and clear thinking they had lost to their opioid habit without even realizing it. Family members thankfully sang my praises. However, I'm afraid my "bias" against opioids and sedatives came out loud and clear to the FRP patients in our failed drug discussions. They told me I was uncaring and prejudiced and just plain not hearing what they had to say.

## DRUG WARS

For a while, I decided to counter this arm wrestling over drugs by sterilizing the FRP drug sessions. The resulting lectures delivered incontrovertible facts about the various classes of medications commonly prescribed to treat back pain. Diagrams depicted the chemical formula for each drug, followed by medical illustrations of the drug's mechanism of action and its anatomic and cellular targets. Terms such as "membrane depolarization" and "spinothalamic tract" come to mind. It didn't take long for the wrangling over opioids to be replaced by the sheer boredom born of all this science talk. Patients were no better informed on how to actually deal with medications, and they rightfully complained. The drug talk was a mess.

One day, the group was especially inattentive, and in desperation I just stopped the lecture and quietly sat down. The room filled with a very awkward feeling that we had come to some sort of crossroad, possibly an impasse. No one wanted to speak first. Finally, I broke the silence with, "What would be helpful for you to know about drugs?"

> Wesley: "Sir, I would like to say that your chemistry talk and the brain picture explain everything, and I'm sure you are correct and stuff, but I don't get what all that has to do with me getting better. You think it would do me any good to take your drawings to my doctor?"

At first, the responses reflected primarily the group's frustration with "all the science stuff" and how that wasn't helpful. They felt the lecture was designed to make me look smart and, in some ways, to justify physicians' authoritarian control over the whole prescription process. "The doctor knows what's good for you" was a promise that had been broken too many times for them to bear. They even implied that doctors protect that control with a cloak of science in order to preserve their billing capacity. For the first time, I began to see from the perspective of people with chronic pain how there could be such a deep distrust of physicians when it came to prescribing drugs. I had been doubly ignorant on this account because I myself had little experience taking prescription medications. However, from my experience as a prescribing physician, I knew all too well how unnerving pain medication discussions could be in the clinic, and I knew that many physicians dreaded this part of caring for people with chronic pain.

## WHAT DO PATIENTS WITH PAIN WANT TO KNOW ABOUT DRUGS?

The FRP participants over the next few months really struggled with the question, "What would be helpful for you to know about drugs?" They felt it was like asking what they would like to know when they didn't know what they needed. The frustration for the patients and for me grew to the point that I gave up trying to assemble the best presentation on what everyone should know about drugs. Just as in the case of learning the critical features of the ideal office visit described in chapter 3, I stopped talking and listened.

I asked one group after another about their experiences with drugs and with the practitioners who prescribed them. I was deeply embarrassed when I admitted to myself that I had neglected a key fact in my previous attempts to make the drug talks useful. Between them, the patients had years of firsthand experience with the very drugs I was expounding on, and they had personal knowledge of the drugs that was far more practical and applicable to themselves as individuals than any generic body of information could ever be.

What I heard completely changed how I talked with and listened to patients about drugs: no more chemical formulas, no more medical illustrations of brains, nerves, and muscles. The groups began to teach me a sensitivity about drugs that I had never really considered. For example, when you put a newly prescribed pill in your mouth, you have no way of knowing what it is going to do to you, for better or for worse. You are depending on the prescriber to predict how the drug will affect you and to assure you that you will not be harmed, often on the basis of a conversation lasting less than a minute. The need for this basic trust can challenge the relationship between patient and prescriber, especially when they are already on shaky ground without a clear diagnosis.

As FRP patients asked me repeatedly to explain how physicians arrive at their drug prescriptions, I had to quiet my own habitual thought patterns in order to clearly hear their stories and understand their questions. The rest of this chapter will take you through the discussion of drugs and medications generated by hundreds of patients relating their experiences and asking for answers to their critical questions.

## EXPERIENCE COUNTS: YOURS!

We begin the session by my going to the whiteboard with black, green, and red markers in hand and asking each patient to call out the names of the medications they have taken or are currently taking for their pain problem. I write the names in black. Some of the names are generic. These are the chemical names, such as acetaminophen, methylprednisolone, and oxycodone. The others are brand names for the same medications: Tylenol, Medrol, and Percodan. Figure 4.1 shows a typical list, with the names gathered into chemical classes of medications. The board always fills up completely before we can write in everyone's list, and the sheer number of drugs astounds the group every time: so many

| OPIOIDS | NSAIDS | ANTI-DEPRESSANTS |
|---|---|---|
| OXYCODONE | IBUPROFEN | AMITRIPTYLINE |
| Percocet | Motrin, Advil | Prozac |
| Roxicet | NAPROXEN | CELEXA |
| Oxycontin | Naprosyn | Citalopram |
| MORPHINE | FELDENE | SERTRALINE |
| CODEINE | RELAFEN | (LITHIUM) |
| HYDROMORPHONE | MOBIC | |
| Dilaudid | Meloxicam | **ANTI-SEIZURE** |
| HYDROCODONE | | GABAPENTIN |
| Vicodin | **STEROIDS** | Neurontin |
| | TRIAMCINOLONE | LYRICA |
| ACETAMINOPHEN | PREDNISONE | |
| Tylenol | Medrol | **ALCOHOL** |
| | | |
| ASPIRIN | **MUSCLE RELAXANTS** | **MARIJUANA** |
| | Flexeril | |
| | METHOCARBAMOL | |
| | Robaxin | |
| | Valium | |

**Figure 4.1.**

different drugs for the single problem of chronic back pain. How can that be? How can we possibly make sense out of all this and develop a strategy for the future?

We first address the group of drugs in the upper left corner by naming them. These are the opioids or narcotics, all chemically related to opium and morphine. Then I ask for each person to describe what, in their own experience, was good about the drug, and I write their responses in green. The list includes "reduces pain" but virtually never "relieves pain." "Takes the edge off" makes the favorites list along with "calms me down." Some members of the group almost always surprise the others by saying these drugs just did not work for them and quickly move on to their intolerance for the sedating effect. "Spacey," "loopy," and "so druggy I couldn't think straight" describe the very quality of calming that other members find so positive. The startled members

| OPIOIDS | NSAIDS | ANTI-DEPRESSANTS |
|---|---|---|
| Less pain | (Little) less pain | Less depressed |
| Takes the edge off | Reduces inflammation? | Calmer |
| *Sedating* | *Heartburn* | *Sedating* |
| *Nausea* | *Upset stomach* | *Dizzy* |
| *Constipation* | *Stomach bleeding* | *Foggy head* |
| *Can't drive* | *Feet swell* | |
| *Addiction* | *Bad for kidneys?* | |
| **MUSCLE RELAXANTS** | **STEROIDS** | **ANTI-SEIZURE** |
| Relaxing | Less pain | Less burn/tingle |
| *Sedating* | *Moody* | *Dizzy* |
| *Can't deal* | *Swollen feet* | *Spacey* |
| **MARIJUANA** | | **ALCOHOL** |
| *Sedating* | | *Sedating* |
| Hurt less | | *Worse afterwards* |
| Don't care so much | | |

**Figure 4.2.**

often look at each other with disbelief, laughing at and sometimes criticizing each other for such disparate responses. I let the conversation evolve as I start writing the negative responses to the drugs in red. Figure 4.2 shows the classes of drugs on the board. Positive effects reported by the group are underlined, and the negative ones are in italics.

Wesley: "Sir, the whole time I was in the first hospital they couldn't figure out why my back and leg hurt so much. They knew I got hurt in combat, so I guess they thought I deserved to be pain free. They gave me more and more 'oxys.' I didn't care about anything. Just as well at first, 'cause I knew some of my buddies didn't make it. By the time they shipped me stateside, I was so hooked. I stayed in bed mostly and, man, was I constipated! Thank God for enemas. No joke, after I finally started shitting, I told them to stop the drugs. And you know what? My pain didn't change that much. I woke up and said to myself in the mirror, 'I got to get out of here, if I'm going to get back to the unit.'"

## DRUGS: ONE SIZE DOES NOT FIT ALL

Quickly, the group reaches the first critical conclusion about drugs: the same drug can have amazingly different effects from one person to the next. Further, the same effect, notably sedation, can be welcome to one person, who may suffer from some degree of anxiety, while deeply troubling to another, who struggles with depression or must stay alert for child care or motor vehicle operation. Chronic opioid users frequently "confess" that while the drug doesn't take away their pain, they just don't care as much about the pain, and they worry less about other parts of their emotional lives. "Things don't bother me so much when I take my meds."

Usually at this point, someone speculates that the differences in drug responses may be related to dosage. "Maybe morphine didn't work for you because you didn't take enough" is suggested alongside "Maybe it made you groggy because you took too much." This line of thinking leads to my asking each person to tell us what dose they have taken of whichever opioid they have experienced. One person says they tried a few doses of 5-mg oxycodone tablets but found that too sedating. Another says they started that way but over time increased their daily dose to more than 100 mg. Again, their looks and laughter express astonishment. How can people have such different appetites for and reactions to the same drug? Sometimes an undercurrent of suspicion creeps into the room. It has to do with an unspoken wondering at what is wrong with the other person that makes them react the way they do. "What makes you need so much 'oxy'?" brings a defensive shrug but no cogent verbal response. Who can say why one person demands a high dose that is unimaginable to someone else? Someone often correlates this uneasiness with the accusative looks they get from medical staff when their office visit comes to a discussion of their opioid use. The patient feels like either a criminal or a crazy person!

## PRESCRIPTION SCIENCE: SKIMPY AT BEST

For a while, I tried to explain drug response differences in scientific terms, such as absorption rates of the drug from the gut into the bloodstream and numbers and modulations of cell membrane drug receptors. I guess I hoped that biological possibilities would diminish the perceived indictments of moral deficiency, perhaps resembling the motivation for some people to call alcohol abuse a disease instead of a psychological fault or turpitude. I gave up on that because these generic biological explanations came across as just educated guesswork and not helpful in any practical way for the individuals in the group.

More important, my efforts to defuse the emotional aspects of the conversation with science distracted the group from another key point: there is no science that tells the prescriber how a given person is going to respond to an opioid for good or bad. The dose at which a given benefit or ill effect will occur is likewise impossible to predict. The group wants to know how doctors choose doses of opioids in the first place, but I ask them to be patient and wait until we can cover more territory on the other drugs. The answers will come by the end of the hour, and they will come both as a surprise and as a relief. There has to be a better way to deal with the prescribing doctor, and there is.

We return to the list of adverse effects the members have experienced with opioids, and to "sedation," already on the board in red and green, the group commonly adds "nausea," "headache," "constipation," and "itching." Most important, they add "addiction."

## ADDICTION

I have given up reporting more formal and official definitions of addiction in favor of listening to the members' own experiences. "I can't live without my pills." "When I try to cut down, I feel like crap." "Once I take my meds, I start thinking about the next time I can take them again." "I get scared and angry when I look in my bottle and there aren't enough pills to get me to the next prescription." Overall, the experience of addiction comes out in terms of real or imagined consequences of not having the drug. Ironically, the opioid veterans in the group rarely talk about addiction as a persisting need for pain relief, presumably the original, positive intent of the prescription. The very word "addiction" brings to mind only negative aspects of the drugs. Recalling the look on the doctor's face when they are requesting opioids, the patients reveal their conclusion that if you are addicted, people suspect there is something either criminally or psychologically wrong with you.

> Wesley: "I guess what happened for me was different from what I saw going on with other guys who told their doctors they had to have their meds. I just got scared that if I didn't stop, I would never get my life back. For me that meant getting back to the unit, to my guys. Maybe I felt a little sick to my stomach and stuff when I quit, but it was worth it to get that fog out of my head. What was really weird was that after a week, I was like, wow, this is me again! I got out of bed and started walking up and down the halls. My back hurt, but my brain was back."

Questions about how the opioids work used to bring me back to the biological explanations that included chemical formulas, brain illustrations, and cell membrane receptors. This didactic response was never satisfying, but it did reveal a profound surprise. What the opioids do not do is fix anything—they do not reduce inflammation or fix the cause of the pain itself. They may take the pain down a notch, but the relief is very rarely complete. Primarily, they just make patients *mind* the pain less. They don't cure anything. Recalling the list of anatomic structures (muscles, bones, ligaments, tendons, and nerves) and mechanisms of injury (strains, sprains, and inflammation) that could possibly be generating their pain from the discussion of the diagnostic process in chapter 3, the patients realize that opioids don't affect any of the spine's potential culprits. Instead, these drugs primarily alter the brain's assessment of the pain without attending to the cause. The group concludes that the opioids are "just band-aids!"

At this point, the group is ready to move on to the next two medications: acetaminophen and aspirin. Each is in a class by itself. Neither is related chemically to the opioids. However, acetaminophen is commonly compounded with the opioids in brand-name products like Percocet and Roxicet ("-cet" is the suffix that means the drug contains acetaminophen). The doses of the drugs are expressed by two numbers separated by a slash. The first number is the opioid dose in milligrams, and the second is the amount of acetaminophen. So, a Percocet 5/325 tablet contains 5 mg of the opioid oxycodone and 325 mg of acetaminophen. I point this out because the maximum safe daily dose of acetaminophen is 3,000 mg, and you have to add up the amount of acetaminophen you are taking mixed into the opioid along with whatever acetaminophen you may be taking independently to make sure you are not overdosing. I make sure everyone remembers the 3,000 number when it comes to drugs with "-cet" in them.

Over the past 30 years, members of the FRP groups have reported less and less use of both aspirin and acetaminophen. In recent years, almost no one has said they have been taking either of these medications on a regular basis. This trend cannot be explained by the well-known potential adverse reactions of these drugs, such as gastrointestinal bleeding or liver toxicity, because the patients do not bring them up as reasons for not taking these medications. Most patients don't consider aspirin or acetaminophen to be capable of serious ill effects because they don't consider these drugs to be potent enough to cause much trouble. Many have tried these medications early in the course of their pain experience but found them to be ineffective and just stopped taking them. Neither of these two drugs merits any mention of good or bad effects from the group: no green or red writing on the board. We do briefly discuss why aspirin's ability to reduce inflammation and the pain-relieving capacity of both drugs might have made them sensible choices. But the patients' experience of inefficacy prevails, so we quickly move on to the next class of medications.

## ANTI-INFLAMMATORY DRUGS

Nonsteroidal anti-inflammatory drugs, so-called NSAIDs, top all the other medications in that virtually everyone has tried at least one. The group calls out so many names, both brand name and generic, that I can't manage the clutter on the board and leave room for the drugs yet to come. Often, ibuprofen, diclofenac, naproxen, and all their associated brand names make the list, but at least 15 others can appear. The faces around the table always reflect the group's "what is going on here?" reaction to the number of available drugs in this class.

Most patients have tried two or three of these drugs, and they tell a common story. Their prescriber has switched them from one drug to another in this class not because there is much known or predictable positive difference but because the new one "might work." The principle of symptom regression to the mean we discussed at length in chapter 3 explains this practice very well. Patients with chronic pain tend to pursue drug changes when their symptoms have worsened, not knowing or believing that their flare-up is very likely to return to baseline on its own. When the new drug has been taken for a week or two (often the time frame the prescriber has predicted the drug will need to have effect) and the patient feels better, both patient and prescriber attribute the recovery to the drug. If repeated, these apparent successes promote a perpetual practice of "trying something new" whenever symptoms worsen.

I ask the group what positive effects they have experienced with the NSAIDs. "Less pain" (albeit limited) and "reduced inflammation" make it to the board in green. The group is careful to clarify that the reduction in pain is very hard to describe or quantify because the drugs do not make them feel buzzed in any way like the opioids do. Without this signal that the drug is doing something, they have a hard time telling what the drug is doing and when to their pain. Veterans of short-acting opioids often have learned that the waning of the sedative effect of the drug in the second half of the dose schedule (say, 3 hours into a 4-hour prescribed interval) heralds a crescendo in their pain. This synchronous association of sedation and pain relief does not happen with the NSAIDs since there is no sedation. Over the years, FRP patient reports of chronic pain relief with NSAIDs have dwindled, and rarely are they now found without supplementation by two or three other medications from the other classes.

The promise of NSAIDs lies in the very name. Although the "NS" part means they are "not steroids" (we will discuss steroids in the next section), the "AI" part stands for "anti-inflammatory," as they are designed to reduce inflammation. So, I ask they group how they know when their backs are inflamed. The resounding reply: "because it hurts!" True enough, pain is the cardinal and most troubling feature of inflammation, but how can they tell the pain is not related to muscle spasm or a strained ligament or a shift of material inside the disc, conditions that don't necessarily involve inflammation? We return briefly to the discussion in chapter 3 and the diagnostic dilemmas of back pain, recalling that the structures capable of hurting in and around the spine are deep beneath the skin and therefore both invisible and untouchable.

Now the three other classical features of acute inflammation come forward. The term "acute" means it comes on quickly in response to injury or invasion by foreign material that is either infectious or toxic in some way. Redness, swelling, and heat are all produced by a complex cavalcade of chemical, cellular, and vascular events that increase blood supply to the area in order to attack any foreign material and start the healing process. When I ask for a description of what happens when you sprain your ankle or are stung by a bee, the responses are uniform: pain, redness, swelling, and heat. So, can you see or feel redness, swelling, or heat in your flared-up back? Of course not, since the structures that are potentially inflamed are too deep beneath the skin to see or touch. You also can't see acute inflammation in these structures with X-ray or magnetic resonance imaging unless there is a rip-roaring infection that has destroyed tissue or created an abscess or sac of pus. Often, the patients say their doctor or therapist told them their backs were inflamed as a rationale for NSAIDs or physical treatments to reduce inflammation. "Come to think of it, how did anybody know there was inflammation going on in there?" They didn't, and it becomes clear to everyone in the group that the prescription of NSAIDs is done purely on speculation with no primary evidence that there is any inflammation going on in the first place.

When I ask the group what doses of these medications they have taken, the response is much more uniform than in the case of the opioids. Unlike opioids, the maximum safe doses of NSAIDs do not vary much between individuals, and these maximums are well established and well known to prescribers.

There just isn't much range from lowest to highest safe dose to choose from. Many of the patients have figured out another practicality of the NSAIDs. In their own experience, there isn't much difference between the various drugs for good or bad, and the dosing rules for taking the over-the-counter standbys ibuprofen and naproxen are right on the label.

So, if the indication for NSAIDs is invisible even if it does exist and the dosing is obvious for inexpensive drugs you can buy without a prescription, who needs a prescription? This is a great question, one we will address at the end of this chapter once we have covered the rest of the drugs.

Wesley: "I had this one doc who told me my pain was nerve pain. This was a few months after I got hurt, when I decided to stop the 'oxys.' He said maybe the nerves were inflamed and we could calm it all down with Motrin. Motrin was like candy to me, and guys told me it was good if you were sore and stuff, like if you overdid it or twisted your ankle. But no way was it gonna do anything for my pain. He was the doctor, not me. But this was no sprain, you know what I mean? So he said we could try a shot of steroids into my back. That sounded scary, but maybe something like, strong, you know, would do something."

## STEROIDS

Almost all FRP patients have had experience with steroids, either in pill form or through injections. The most common pills are prednisone (more than 80 brand names) and methylprednisolone (brand name Medrol), coming in a plastic pack enclosing the pills for each day in tapering columns. While some patients describe mood changes, upset stomach, and occasionally swollen feet, which I record in red on the board, most don't report negative side effects. Unfortunately, reports of success from these patients with chronic pain are rare and are usually complicated by the patient's having taken other drugs at the same time. Response to my request for something to write in green comes vaguely, but most of the group members recall they were told that the steroid was meant to reduce inflammation and that it was stronger than the NSAID they might have tried already. Everyone seems to have been told that you can't take these drugs for long without running the risk of weakening of your bones through osteoporosis.

Patients who have chief complaints of leg or arm pain have commonly had epidural injections of liquid steroids into the epidural space surrounding the nerve roots as they exit the spine. Recalling the anatomy lessons of chapter 3, perhaps the most classical explanation for sciatica since the 1930s has been a piece of disc poking through its back wall and irritating and inflaming a nerve root along its egress out of the spine toward the leg. This inflamed nerve root is the target of epidural injections, though there is virtually never any inflammation evident to patient or provider. Others have had steroids injected into or near multiple facet joints. Recall that these joints resemble the last joint in your finger, and you have a pair of them between the backsides of the vertebra above and the one below at each segment of your spine. They are progressively affected by osteoarthritis through the decades of life whether you have back pain or not. The same can be said for the sacroiliac joints, which connect your sacrum (the flat bone down below your belt line in back), and the pelvic bones, which go out to both sides toward your hips. The sacroiliac joints can be painfully inflamed by diseases like ankylosing spondylitis, but hardly any FRP patients have these conditions.

Most of the patients have tried combinations of these injections into the spine and joints, although some cringe at the idea of being stuck in their back or neck and wouldn't dream of letting anyone near them with a needle. Hundreds of patients recounting how they ended up getting injected and into which targets have at times led the groups to wonder what the heck is going on here. Reports of clearly indicated and understood rationales for the injections, such as disc herniation and resulting acute nerve root inflammation, constitute a small fraction of all these procedures. Many of the patients have "been through the mill," from one injection to the next in hopes of finding the true target and reducing inflammation that cannot possibly be demonstrated in any event. The fact that all these injectable medications last for only a matter of days makes them unlikely candidates for success in curing conditions that have gone on for months or years, but hope springs eternal, especially when there is a flare-up that the patient just can't tolerate.

## MUSCLE RELAXANTS

"Back spasm" plausibly explains back pain in the minds of many medical practitioners and back pain patients alike. Many FRP participants have been told—and some believe—that spasm is to blame for their flare-ups. In medical terms, "spasm" means the sustained contraction of a muscle that has not been initiated intentionally. Spinal cord injuries can cause true, sustained spasms in the muscles supplied by nerves that exit the cord below the injury. Neuromuscular diseases, such as multiple sclerosis, can also produce muscular spasm. But people don't really consider those more serious forms of spasm when they talk about their back pain. They are thinking more along the lines of a "charley horse" or the painful tightening of a calf muscle that wakes you in the night. And they are thinking that this kind of spasm can go on for days or weeks.

Another type of muscular contraction commonly claimed to be the cause of back and neck pain is a less dramatic and more chronic contraction of muscles associated with emotional stress. FRP patients with chronic neck pain frequently report catching themselves in stressful situations and noticing that their neck and shoulder muscles have drawn their shoulders up toward their ears. Some have learned that by looking into the mirror and taking slow, deep breaths, they can lower their shoulders and get some relief.

Whether members of the group believe their back pain is the result of true spasm or stress-related chronic contraction, the idea of relaxing the muscles makes sense to them and to their health care providers as well. Most FRP patients have been told by one practitioner or another, especially by physical and massage therapists, that their muscles are tight, even in spasm. So, rubbing and stretching the muscles make sense. While there are various beliefs and theories about pain being caused by the contraction of tiny muscles, by far the most common concept among FRP patients over the years has involved what they perceive as the big muscles alongside the lower spine. "Even my wife can feel those muscles in spasm when my back goes out." Similar reports frequently provoke the following exercise.

## MUSCLE SPASM?

I ask everyone to stand up and do what I do. With my back turned toward them, I stand on my right foot and shift my pelvis a little to the right. I place my palms over my lower back so that the fingertips of each hand are almost touching those of the other hand, elbows out to the side. "What do you feel?" The uniform response: "The big muscles on the right are bigger and harder, just like when I am in spasm." Then I ask them to shift their weight and pelvis to the left, keeping their hands in place. Presto! The "spasm" disappears on the right and spreads to the muscles on the left. Many patients experiencing this shift have told me this exercise totally debunked their concept of spasm. I can conclude only that many patients and practitioners mistake small, often involuntary shifts in spinal alignment to avoid compression or strain of painful tissues for spasm, and they proceed to the treatment of spasm.

As controversial as the diagnosis of muscle spasm may be, drugs to relax muscles sit in the medicine cabinets of most FRP patients whether they are using them or not. So, I ask what has been good about the drugs in their own experience, and I write the common response in green on the board: "They relax!" Almost no one over the years has said they relax muscles. Rather, they relax the person or at least make the person less anxious about their pain. "What has been bad about them?" brings "sedation," "groggy," and the like. Just as with the opioids, one person's positive calming effect is another's foggy nap.

Once again, we have a class of mediations whose biological target is vague and rarely diagnosed with clinical objectivity and whose effects cannot be predicted by the prescriber. The FRP patients have reported a wide variety of responses to these drugs over the years, but a definite pattern has emerged. People whose pain experience includes anxiety commonly seek relief from that component with medications, and the muscle relaxants and benzodiazepines remain popular options. But the goal of blunting the worries that go with chronic pain has been increasingly addressed with opioids, even though patients generally speak with their prescribers about the need for pain relief from these drugs, feeling that mention of the antianxiety effect will be frowned on as an illegitimate indication.

## ALCOHOL AND MARIJUANA

When the groups discuss "relaxing" drugs, I ask them what substances are most commonly used to this end in our society. Sometimes they need a little prompting because the answers are not on the board yet. The assenting "aha" and "oh, yeah" come when someone blurts out "alcohol" and another "marijuana." I'm not sure why, but someone generally cracks a joke about "booze" or makes a sucking sound holding a pretend joint to their lips. Almost everyone has used alcohol at some point (and many chronically) to soften the blows of their pain and anxiety, especially at night, when alcohol can help some people get to sleep. Reports of alcohol actually reducing pain are rare, but some people do say drinking can "take the edge off," referring to the mental numbing effect. Again, the results vary tremendously and unpredictably from one individual to the next. Because alcohol is readily available without prescription and people in general are familiar with safe dosage, people with chronic pain commonly experiment with alcohol as a form of self-treatment. Over the years, FRP participants have occasionally reported some benefit from alcohol, often in the context of drinking themselves to sleep, but hardly anyone claims alcohol to be effective in treating their pain. On the contrary, stories of alcohol making their lives even more miserable and complicated abound.

Marijuana shares with alcohol this vast range and variety of responses, and its unpredictability of the results for a given individual exceeds that of alcohol. FRP patients in the early years rarely brought out their experience with marijuana, partly because it was illegal. More important, the potency of commonly available marijuana was reportedly insufficient to have much positive effect. Through the years, participants have grown more comfortable talking about marijuana, but again the resounding message has been that one man's positive potion is another's poison. While some people report blunting of their pain experience, others find it actually enhances the pain, perhaps by intensifying their attention to the pain.

In wrapping up our discussion of alcohol and marijuana, I ask the groups to consider any potential curative effect these substances might have. While almost everyone assumes that these drugs work on the brain, no one has much knowledge about their biochemical effects, and no one suspects that they are fixing the source of their pain in any way. This realization that whatever the drugs are doing takes place in the brain brings us logically to the last two classes of medications: antiseizure and antidepressant drugs.

## IS THE PAIN IN YOUR BRAIN?

If it hasn't already come up, right about here in the session someone brings up the question, "So, Doctor, are you saying my pain is all in my head?" I quickly respond that I don't know and that I gave up trying to answer that question for individual patients a long time ago. In a perfect world, medical providers would be able to parse out how much of an individual's pain came from a physical source in the body and how much resulted from some process in the brain. Their prescriptions would be informed by this incrimination of mind versus body.

> Wesley: "Sir, I just never could get into it when they told me Neurontin was for seizures. Like, I saw a guy have a seizure once, and no way was my problem like that. I guess that doesn't make sense to think like that, but I just knew it was not going to work. I took it though for months, and then I stopped it by myself, even though they told me not to 'cause it might be working, and I just didn't know it. Well, my leg didn't feel any different without out the meds, so I guess it was like I was my own doctor now. Maybe that's crazy, but it's what happened to me."

For some years, I tried speaking in science-based parables that began with stepping on a tack. The stories described how even if the tack were removed and the punctured tissues healed, the pain could remain for months and years. I tried talking about ways in which pain signals might persist for some reason in taking nerve pathways leading from the site of the pain up through the spinal cord to centers in the brain where they could be interpreted, creating emotive and behavioral reactions. I talked about neuroplasticity, using analogies like the brain consisting of millions of vinyl records whose grooves could be rerouted or even created anew. I described the historical shift from assuming one is born with a finite number of brain cells that inexorably diminish over time to the discovery that the brain is constantly changing by generating new nerve cells and pathways. As much as I studied what was being discovered and published about brain mechanisms of changing, especially in the area of interpreting pain, I had to admit I didn't really know what I was talking about in any way that made much of an impression on the FRP groups.

It took a while for my frustration to teach me to stop explaining and start listening. Time to take my own medicine again. I began paying more attention to what the FRP groups were telling me to write on the board both in green and in red regarding antiseizure and antidepressant drugs. The patterns of positive and negative effects were so consistent that I was embarrassed I hadn't understood or even recognized them before.

The words in red came quickly from people who had suffered the sedation and mental numbing or dizziness common to these drugs. Usually, these ill effects came on suddenly soon after beginning to take these medications and were easily relieved by stopping the drug. Because of this immediate association, patients did not have trouble identifying the drug as the culprit.

The words in green were sparse and weak. Most of the time, there were none. While some people said their pain was maybe better when they started taking gabapentin (brand name Neurontin, an antiseizure medication) or any of the antidepressants, it was hard for them to know if the drug was making this difference. Certainly, whatever positive effect the medication might have had on the pain was less than dramatic. The most common prescriptions for gabapentin began with low doses building up to the point where patients were either getting side effects or believing that they were feeling less pain because of the drug. This titration process might have taken weeks, making it even more difficult to know whether to credit the drug for the improvement. One way to test whether a drug is working after taking it for a long time is to stop it. However, that approach is not feasible with gabapentin because safe cessation requires gradual tapering. Suddenly stopping it can be dangerous. Knowing that your pain can wax and wane on its own in a matter of days or weeks can make assessment of a drug's efficacy a real problem when the drug has to be started and stopped over a similar time frame.

One thing is for sure about the positive effects of antiseizure and antidepressant medications: only the person taking the medication has any real chance of knowing whether it is doing them any good. These drugs do not have any objective effect that can be measured by an outside observer. There is no relevant blood test or any practical imaging available in common clinical situations. Whatever the drugs are doing in the brain or spinal cord cannot be observed in any practical way. A possible exception to this rule has to do with the "look in the eye" and facial expressions called "affect" in medical jargon in people who are depressed. Sometimes, when such a person starts taking an antidepressant medication, medical providers, even family members and acquaintances, notice a definite "brightening" of the person's affect as if "the lights are back on."

As the hour draws to a close, the groups always want to know what to take away from what has generally been a discouraging discussion. I acknowledge their frustration and ask them to consider what we have concluded from their own experience:

- The prescription of medications for chronic back pain is almost never based on an objective diagnosis of a biological target, such as inflammation of a joint or involuntary contraction of a muscle.
- Because there is no objective target, drug effects are subjective. Only the person who is taking the drug can tell what effect the drug is having on him or her.
- Prescribers are not able to reliably predict what effect a given drug is going to have on an individual—for good or for bad.
- Patients with chronic back pain often end up taking several different medications, making it difficult to know which one is having what effect.

How can we integrate these conclusions with our observations from prior chapters about the challenges of communicating unmeasurable symptoms, setting personal goals, and optimizing the medical office visit and decision making? Can we get past the visit in which a brief and unrewarding discussion of symptoms and tests leads only to a contentious negotiation over prescription drugs? Absolutely, we can. Hopefully, this chapter and the preceding one have laid the groundwork for people with chronic back pain and their medical providers to establish and maintain relationships that mutually satisfy. The key to this success lies in a shared understanding of what life goals really matter to the person in pain and in focusing on achieving those goals. Drug prescription in this context is rarely contentious. This approach will come as a shock to those in pain and their caregivers who have long insisted that the pursuit of a happy life can begin only when they have found the right drug to remove the pain.

Once you and your doctor have settled on the best regimen for you, stick with it through your 21-day training program. Changing drugs or their doses during progressive exercise can be very confusing should your pain get better or worse. You won't be able to tell whether the ups and downs with your pain are due to the increasing activity or to the new pill or different dose. Should your goals require cessation of pain or anxiety medications, make the change before or after your program. If your back has given you enough trouble that you need the 21-day program, chances are excellent that you are going to continue to experience fluctuating pain during your training. So, you are going to need some nondrug skills to deal with the pain and your worries. The next two chapters aim to give you effective coping tools: deep relaxation and physical self-care for painful flare-ups.

## • 5 •

# Relaxation

$\mathcal{S}$tressed and depressed—hardly anyone disabled by chronic back pain isn't one or both. Certainly, interviews and questionnaires have consistently revealed high levels of both conditions in patients participating in functional restoration programs (FRPs) over the past three decades. While the debate rages on as to whether these emotional states cause pain or vice versa, there can be no doubt that they contribute to the patients' overall suffering and stifle their efforts to recover physical function and active lifestyles. What to do about these pervasive complicators of chronic pain? How to present any intervention without implying that "the pain is all in your head"? These two questions have driven FRPs through a long and tortuous quest for the most practical and effective skills that the patients can take with them going forward with their lives.

### ROBERT

Across the classroom table from you sits 52-year-old Robert. His tattooed, wiry arms, shoulder-length hair, and shaggy beard make you wonder if he isn't a biker or maybe a mountain man. In fact, he has been a live-alone roofer all his adult life—that is, until he fell off a roof 2 years ago. The ambulance crew reported he must have landed on his feet, and he did fracture a bone above his right ankle. He only knows that when he came to in the hospital the next day, his back hurt more than his ankle. His fracture eventually healed up all right, but he couldn't understand why his back kept hurting so

85

much when his doctors told him his X-rays and magnetic resonance imaging scan showed "there's nothing wrong with your spine." As the months went by, though, his back was not his biggest problem. He was terrified of getting back on a roof.

Today's FRP session begins with a question to the group: "What words come to mind when I say the word, 'relaxation'?" "Poolside," "cocktails," "sitting by the fire," "the beach," and "vacation" are common responses. I announce that the relaxation we are going to talk about is not related to any of those things. I admit that talking about relaxation is like talking about singing. Talking about singing is not like singing. To learn how to sing, you have to actually *sing*. "Relax!" I blurt out. Half of the group is stunned; the others start laughing. I briefly confess that they won't learn how to relax in a way that can truly help them by my *talking* about relaxation, nor can they expect to reap relaxation's benefits by *trying* to relax a few times. Often, some members of the group have had lots of experience with yoga, meditation, and various other forms of relaxation. Others consider the topic some kind of psycho voodoo related to hippies and gurus and Eastern religions. Hopefully, today's discussion can enlist their prior experiences and attitudes in forming a personally effective tool for dealing with stress.

## HOW BRAINS WORK: COMA

I step up to the whiteboard and ask the group, "What is the lowest level your brain can function at and you can still be alive?" "Coma" is an immediate response almost every time. Often, someone introduces the concept of brain death and the role of "brain wave tests" or electroencephalography (EEG) in detecting brain function. I ask them to assume that there is at least something going on in the comatose person's mind. So, what is it about a person that makes us say he or she is in a coma? "They're unconscious" and "They don't respond" are two answers that prompt the question of what they are unconscious of or not responding to. Sometimes the group includes a nurse or other medical person who has experience in intensive care units where patients' lives are supported by breathing machines called ventilators and pumps to keep their blood circulating. These providers report that the comatose patient does not respond to sound ("Can you hear me?"), pain (pinching a finger or rubbing the sternum), light (a flashlight shown in the eye), or smell (coffee under the nose). Okay, so in the most basic way of thinking about coma, we may not be able to tell if an unconscious person is thinking or not, but we say the person is comatose when he or she doesn't react to common stimuli in any demonstrative way. So I write "Coma" in the upper left hand corner of the board and ask the group for the next higher state of mind or level of brain function.

## SLEEP

Insomnia is so rampant among people with chronic pain that this part of the brain discussion always starts with "How can we get *more* sleep?" I ask the group to hold on to that question until later in the hour, when they can answer it for themselves. For now, I write "Sleep" just to the right of "Coma" on the board. We turn to the difference between sleep and coma. Everyone knows that unlike the person in a coma, a sleeping person you can wake up. Sometimes it is harder to wake them up than others, and people, especially those who have experience with arousing sleeping children or snoring spouses, know that some stages of sleep are "deeper" than others. We used to have quite technical discussions of the depths or stages of sleep, including such topics as rapid eye movement and dream states, but they just weren't helpful in any practical way, so we deleted them. They were another example of lessons the FRP staff and I thought the patients should learn but held no interest or value for the patients. Without dwelling further on the nature of sleep, I ask the group for the next higher level of consciousness.

> Robert: "I've always had trouble falling asleep. A few beers after dinner used to help. Now even a six-pack doesn't work. I just lie there thinking about my back. What am I supposed to do if I can't work?"

## BEING AWAKE

This question generates a mixture of quizzical and stumped looks around the table. As I write "Awake" to the right of "Sleep," everyone agrees that we are all awake, but what is it like? How is it different from being asleep? I tell the group that in my perception, what I have been saying is *so fascinating* that they have been paying attention to the sound of my voice. But what other noises have been going on since the session began? There is a clock ticking at the end of the room. The heating and ventilation system has been very lightly humming overhead. A few voices have been heard coming from people passing by in the hallway on the other side of the wall. Members of the group differ surprisingly in what sounds they have been aware of, but everyone recognizes that they have somehow easily extinguished their attention to these sounds in order to come back to the voices in our conversation.

What else has been going on during the session so far? How about the sensation in your right foot as it rests in your shoe on the floor? What about the color of my shirt? What does the air feel like on your face and in your nostrils as you breathe? How about the smells in the room? How has your back been feeling with all this sitting? How many of you have had at least one thought about something going on outside of this room and unrelated to this conversation pass through your mind since the session began? Everyone raises their hand.

Once we have reviewed the above sensory and thought experiences, every group comes to the conclusion that seeing, hearing, smelling, and tasting; feeling pain, pressure, and temperature; and the capacity to let go of distractions and *focus* on one sensation at a time critically characterize the brain state we call being awake. "Awareness" and "attention" are words that commonly come up here. Now comes the group's effort to describe the level of brain work above the sensing and thinking we have been doing while we have been awake.

## HYPER

Through the years, the FRP groups have described this state of mind with words like "anxious," "afraid," "wired," "worried," and "stressed out." Everyone knows what we are talking about, so I ask them to describe what sensations occur in their bodies when they have these feelings. I write their list below the word "Hyper": breathing faster, heartbeat goes up, blood pressure goes up, and tension mounts in the muscles, the only body parts that *can* get tense. Further entries often include queasy stomach ("butterflies") and lightheadedness.

> Robert: "A lot of guys I used to work with would get the jitters when they got to the work site. They would have a liquid breakfast or blow a joint before they went up on the roof. Not me. I saw them make too many stupid mistakes. All my life I figured if you fall, you fall. Until I fell."

Someone in the group knows that this reaction and these bodily sensations are produced when the brain and the part of the nervous system called the "sympathetic" nervous system release a surge of adrenaline. Although the name of this chemical sounds familiar, rarely does anyone know how it works. Somehow the knowledge that this reaction they have felt for themselves is a *physical reality* is validating, so they want to know how it works. I explain that adrenaline is a chemical released by one nerve cell to attach to its neighbor to make that next cell fire off a message to its neighbors. This neuro-messaging is happening billions of times a second throughout the body. It is normally going on in the counterbalancing part of the nervous system, called the "parasympathetic" nervous system, but not when the sympathetic surge takes over.

## FIGHT OR FLIGHT

Now comes the question of what could possibly be the reason for something stressful to trigger this immediate flow of adrenaline throughout the body. Invariably, someone in the group blurts out, "Fight or flight." Correct. So, why would it be useful for you to breathe faster and for your heart to beat faster, your blood pressure to go up, and your muscles to tense up? "So you can run away or stand and fight." Correct. The purpose of all this adrenaline and its bodily effects is to get oxygen into your blood and send it to your muscles so they can go to work.

This is all making sense to the group. So, I ask them what situations in real life would require muscular performance without even pausing to think things over. This request virtually always stumps the group, and I let the silence linger to make a point. "How about if you were walking through the jungle, and a tiger jumped out in front of you?" "How about if you just thought you saw the tail of a tiger behind a rock?" These scenarios bring out varieties of "Run for your life." "How about walking down a dark alley, and someone jumps out in front of you?" That seems more likely and a very good reason to make a run for it. But the groups can almost never come up with other situations where this fight-or-flight reaction is useful in real life.

Occasionally, there is a former athlete who talks about the reaction building up as a game or race is about to begin and describes the need to calm down the emotional motivation in order to take advantage of the physical response and perform well. A firefighter may describe what it feels like right before breaking into a burning house.

## WHAT TROUBLES YOU?

I ask the group to think about their own lives and what events or situations actually make them anxious, worried, or fearful. What makes them go from "Awake" to "Hyper"? Every time, money tops the list. "Bills," "credit cards," "car payments," "taxes," and the like are common concerns that represent at some level a threat to survival. It's not the money itself that's the problem; rather, it's the fear of destitution that comes from not having it. In our consumer, money-based society, this fear runs rampant. Right behind money come work and family. Work generates anxiety in two primary ways. First, the ubiquitous fear of losing your job makes everyone nervous because unemployment clearly threatens survival and, perhaps more subtly, self-esteem. Second, squabbles with coworkers often turn out to be more about respect than factual content. Family issues include interspousal arguments and the aggravating things that kids do. Virtually every member of every FRP group suffers from these family "issues." The FRP groups consistently report that money and sex generate most spousal spats. The ensuing discussion always leads to their conclusion that deep down these flare-ups create fear of losing love and the feeling of belonging or *connection.* Worries over sickness and especially symptoms that might mean cancer make the list, but two fears that you would logically expect to come out on top do not. Over several years of my asking for real-life causes of anxiety, fear of dying has never come up. But the most striking absentee is pain. Pain makes the list from about 1 in 10 groups. I cannot say why this happens, and I'm always surprised when it does. For every group that omits pain, I ask why they didn't bring it up. In general, they explain that pain just does not carry the same kind of emotional weight as do money, work, and family feuds. Pain is also somehow different from sickness, disease, and death. In the end, though, every group concedes that pain *should* go on the list if only because of the fear factors involved.

Figure 5.1 shows the board as it has developed so far. I now ask the group to reconsider the fight-or-flight response. "How useful are pumped-up muscles in dealing with the items on your real-life worries list?" It is obvious to all that the fight-or-flight reaction to everyday stressors is not only inappropriate and ineffective but also very likely to be counterproductive. Responding to a provocative spouse or child with your muscles is not going to turn out well. The same is true for disagreements with your coworker or boss. Fighting or running away won't help you balance your bank account or pay off your credit cards.

| COMA | SLEEP | AWAKE | HYPER |
|------|-------|-------|-------|
| | | | Adrenaline |
| | | | |
| | | $ | FIGHT/FLIGHT |
| | | Family | ^ Breathing |
| | | Spouse/kids | ^ Heart rate |
| | | Work | ^ Blood pressure |
| | | Boss/co-workers | |
| | | Sex | ^ Muscles!! |
| | | Sickness | |

**Figure 5.1.**

## LIFE IS TROUBLE

What if all the stressors on our list just went away? Everyone laughs at this question. No one believes his life will ever be free of these troubles. Work, money, family, and disease are just plain part of life. Not only do these issues enter every life, but they also challenge us in fact or in our thoughts every day and night. No one has any problem recognizing that some degree of anxiety and the resulting fight-or-flight sensations can come over us at any time and in any place. You can't avoid troubles and worries, but you can try to escape. And do we ever try!

When the group considers the brain states, the fight-or-flight notes, and the list of stressors on the board, represented in figure 5.1, we are ready to talk about ways to stop the pathway through which life drives people from "Awake" to "Hyper" and the fight-or-flight response. I draw an arrow representing this pathway and ask the group what can be done to block the stressors from creating the emotional and physiological consequences.

## COUNSELING

Many of the FRP participants have already had one or more courses of psychotherapy, and their stories in this session reflect the vast diversity of treatments out there in the professional counseling world when it comes to a chief complaint of chronic pain. One point comes through loud and clear: you have no idea what you are going to get when you call the counselor's office to make your first appointment. When a well-meaning primary care provider or claim manager suggests counseling, some people jump to the "all in my head" conclusion and never follow up. The stigma of mental illness and the suggestion that you must have chronic pain because you are a bad or inadequate person forge strong barriers to accepting the vulnerability required for real participation in counseling. Would you bare your soul to someone you don't know in the context of the mess you are in, a mess that the medical profession has not fixed in any way? Yes, if you are desperate. No, if you don't believe you are crazy.

Robert: "You wouldn't believe this one guy I went to. Since I fell, I am totally fucked up about going up on a roof again. This guy said he could fix me. His deal was he would have me lie down on a table, and he would kind of whisper stuff in my ear. Stuff like, 'you are feeling calm' and 'you are brave and strong.' I got out of there as fast as I could. It was creepy."

Depending on how much time we have in the session and what the group's interest may be, I talk briefly about efforts we have made over the years in FRPs to reduce stress reactions and improve moods through counseling. Everyone involved in developing the early FRPs acknowledged that, chickens or eggs, pain and stress and depression often arrived hand in hand. We also knew how stress and depression could impede a person's functional recovery, even their participation in the program. To combat these impediments, early FRPs offered some combination of group and individual counseling incorporating rationalization, shifting the locus of control, analytical inventory, and collective venting, all of which will be explained below. The patients started every program by completing anxiety and depression questionnaires, and we kept careful track of their test results throughout the programs and into the follow-up years. We wanted to know if what we were doing was having any real impact on these all-important aspects of the patients' lives.

## RATIONAL EMOTIVE THERAPY

Albert Ellis was an American psychologist who proposed, starting in the 1950s, that human mental suffering came largely by a pathway from beliefs about life events leading to thoughts, emotions, and behaviors. What beliefs and attitudes you brought to a given experience determined what thoughts and emotions you would experience and what responsive action you would take. This model seemed to be an accurate fit with the chronic pain patient's fear of reinjury. If a person believed that his sudden flare-up of pain resulted from his own stupidity in taking out the trash, an act that had caused pain before, he might berate himself and vow never to take out the trash again.

For years, we led FRP patients through group and individual sessions of examining the reality, the *rationality*, of their thinking. We often taught these lessons through scenarios. Let's say you are walking down the sidewalk, and you see a good friend coming along. You wave and say hello, but he passes you by without a word. You spend the next few days wondering what you might have said or done recently to turn him off. You seem to remember he didn't thank you after the party you threw for his birthday. Sometimes he doesn't return your calls. All these thoughts boil up into an angry steam. Damned if you are ever going to call him again. What a jerk! Two days later, he calls you to announce his mother's death. He has been in a total funk for a week. He has hardly been able to eat or sleep. He never even saw you on the sidewalk.

A 65-year-old man notices his urinary stream is dwindling. He is sure this means he has prostate cancer, just like his uncle did. His uncle died. He is terrified. He stays home for days ruminating about all the things he didn't accomplish in his life. How would he have felt and what would he have done if he had believed his diminishing pee was just a matter of getting older? An accepting shrug?

Stories like this can be helpful in getting people to stop jumping to unproductive, even harmful conclusions when an event throws them into a tizzy. Rational emotive therapy aims to help people break the habit of reacting to events with anxiety, fear, and depression by examining their beliefs and thoughts about the events in more rational ways, leading to more positive actions and outcomes. You will learn more about this approach when we discuss acute and chronic pain in chapter 6.

> Robert: "I just can't believe how messed up I am about going back up on the roof. It used to mean nothing to me. I've been up on thousands of roofs, but no way now! Call me a chicken, but I'm not going back up there."

## LOCUS OF CONTROL

Who or what is responsible for what takes place in your life? If you believe that life pretty much happens to you and that you have no control or determination, the basic FRP business of setting goals and working hard to achieve them will not work for you. As the paradigm of goal achievement became an imperative in the programs, counseling in the programs focused more and more on encouraging patients to take responsibility for their lives. While this approach made sense, over time it became clear that patients were not having much luck shifting their locus of control from the outside to the inside. Once again, listening to the patients taught us what was going on. This form of therapy felt to them like they were being told what to do—what they *should* do because it was *good for them*. Locus of control–based counseling was just too authoritarian, too top-down, to be accepted.


## GROUP THERAPY


In the early years of FRPs, many days ended with the patients sitting together and talking about their experiences. A staff facilitator with psychological training encouraged participants to air their feelings. Otherwise, there was no agenda. These meetings tended to develop into gripe sessions, especially when one or more of the group members were struggling with the training program. Personalities clashed. Feathers flew. The facilitator was frequently challenged to keep the peace. We had hoped that these meetings would provide a chance for group members to get their feelings out in the open and experience together and individually a kind of catharsis. While there were occasional wins, most of the sessions put participants and staff in uneasy if not frankly negative moods.


## INDIVIDUAL TALK THERAPY


The counseling staff were well aware that people disabled by chronic pain carry heavier burdens of depression and anxiety than their peers without pain. Certainly, the FRP patients' scores on admission mood-related questionnaires gave ample evidence of psychological problems. Interviews commonly revealed personal histories of physical and emotional abuse during childhood. Patients frequently reported discord at home, and the staff became particularly challenged in dealing with family members who appeared to be enabling or even supporting the patient's disability. All these issues were addressed in one-on-one counseling sessions throughout many years of the FRPs. These appointments were built into the patient's daily training schedule. It was not uncommon for a session to close at a particularly emotional moment. In tears, the patient would return to the group in the gym, too stressed out to participate. Overall, individual counseling helped some patients, but short-term insight therapy had its limitations.

> Robert: "I was so pissed off in the group yesterday, I couldn't even talk. I felt like my head would pop. I worked hard my whole life so I could get away from all the crap that happened to me as a kid. Now the scenes keep coming back into my head. I am such a piece of shit."

## COUNSELING COMES TO AN END

The demise of formal psychological counseling came not from careful consideration but rather through an experiment of nature. Lack of insurance reimbursement for psychological services eventually forced their discontinuation. Thereafter, we continued to monitor the patients' results on the mood-related questionnaires, only to find that their scores actually improved. Discussions with program graduates and review of their 1-year follow-up questionnaires revealed their own insights that mood improvement came not as much from resolution of stressors as from a general feeling of well-being due to increasing physical exercise and overcoming personal pain-related phobias and self-impairment. You will see how this appreciation for the psychological impact of exercise eventually led to the program's focus on wellness in chapter 7.

## COUNSELING VERSUS RELAXATION

After reviewing the above counseling approaches and the "Coma"–"Sleep"–"Awake"–"Hyper" scheme, today's FRP group is finally ready to discuss relaxation. I return to the board and suggest that there is an alternative to the pathway through which life's stressors drive people from "Awake" to "Hyper." I suggest that there is a state of mind we have not yet put on the board, and that state is relaxation. I write "Relaxation" on the board. I ask if any of the group's members who have had experience with relaxation techniques prior to attending the current program can describe what relaxation is like to the rest of us. It is often fascinating, sometimes amusing, to witness the word wrestling that ensues. The short list of positive descriptors is limited to rather bland words, like "calm" and "peaceful." The other members grow restless as I sit there in silence. Finally, I thank the members who tried to describe what relaxation "feels" like and acknowledge that *talking* about relaxation is challenging indeed.

## RELAXATION TECHNIQUES

By this time in the program, the participants have had a session or two of each of the following approaches to relaxation. Progressive muscle contraction and relaxation begins with lying down or sitting and squeezing your feet as if you were a bird clasping something with your talons. You hold the squeeze for a few seconds, then release. You repeat this contraction and release a few times. Next, you complete a similar cycle with your calf muscles, your thigh muscles, your buttocks, your lower back, your belly, your chest, your hands, your forearms, your shoulders, your jaw, your mouth, and your face around your eyes.

Visualization involves listening to a recording of someone describing a peaceful scene, such as a garden path or a beach. The voice encourages you to imagine yourself walking along. You may hear birds chirping, the wind caressing the trees, and the waves breaking on the shore. You may happen on a small box on a post. You are invited to stop, put your troubles into the box, then walk along unburdened.

Tai chi and yoga are two ancient methods that combine movement and posture with breathing and focusing. Mindfulness-based stress reduction centers on the breath while maintaining a form of awareness that can be summarized with the saying, "I am breathing in. I am breathing out." Sometimes there is a Catholic in the group who has experience with the Rosary and repetitive prayer.

Years ago, I gave up on trying to explain the historical backgrounds of these various techniques. I also quit talking about the scientific discoveries of their physiological effects, such as lowering blood pressure and heart rate, boosting the immune system, and improving mood through enhancing dopamine "flow" in the brain. Group after group reported that my attempts to validate the techniques were not only unconvincing but also boring. Time for me to listen again.

## RELAXATION: ONE SIZE DOES NOT FIT ALL

So, I ask the group members to raise their hands if they have tried visualization. Everyone does so. "Who feels they became really deeply relaxed?" Three things almost always happen here. One or two people raise their hands, the rest do not, and a few people start laughing. The laughter comes from people who report that one of the group fell asleep during the visualization session and snored so loudly they had to be nudged awake. I ask the group to remember this moment when we talk about the difference between sleep and relaxation and how to take advantage of it. I ask the people who did not raise their hands what happened. "I just couldn't get into it." "The lady's voice drove me crazy." "I couldn't stop thinking about my back pain." "I just wanted it to be over so we could have lunch." I ask those who raised their hands what the relaxed state felt like. They are just as stumped as the relaxation veterans were in the beginning of the class. "Calm" and "peaceful" come up again but not "sleepy."

I lead the group through the same exercise, reviewing their experience with progressive muscle contraction and relaxation. No one reports that they fell asleep, but they have experienced the same disparity in relaxation results. When I ask the group what they think is the *best* technique for relaxation, the conclusion is unanimous. Each person has his or her own favorite, and there is no rhyme or reason to it. Further, no one could have predicted which technique would work for them ahead of time. You have to try these methods to know for yourself what works for you. Somehow this realization is far more powerful in convincing people to practice relaxation than all the explaining I used to do.

## PRACTICE MAKES PERFECT

Now is the time to push the "practice" button. I explain to the group that relaxation is a skill. By that, I mean you get good at it by doing it over and over until you can perform it consistently and effectively even when you are under duress. You are not going to get good at high diving by reading about it or trying it once or twice. When it's time to compete and it's your turn up there on the platform with all those people looking up at you, you have a much better chance of a safe, clean dive if you have done that dive many, many times and you know in your heart that *you've got this.*

Which method should you practice? The one that works best for *you.* How do you know which one is best for you? You try different techniques until you find one that makes you relax, even if it only relaxes you a little bit. You are probably not going to hit a home run on the first try.

At this point, the group wants to know what key features these techniques may have in common. They also want to know how they are supposed to "relax" when they return to their "real" worlds. As it turns out, these two questions have the same answers.

## HOW TO RELAX

"When you have felt deeply relaxed, what was going on around you?" The response to my question is always the same: "Nothing really, unless I was listening to a tape. The room was quiet, and I had my eyes closed." Everyone easily agrees that the critical component of relaxation is that, beyond your point of focus, your space is quiet. So, I write "Quiet" on the board. Rock music, partying, or watching football on TV may give you a boost and wind down into a sense of fatigue, but that is not what we are shooting for here.

"So what was going on in your mind?" "I was focusing on my breathing." "I was paying attention to my breath." "I was just feeling my muscles squeeze and release." Right, so I write "Focus" on the board. Underneath, I write "Breathing" because most focusing methods involve paying attention to your breath. You can count upward to a target number while you inhale and back down while you are breathing out. You can say something positive as you breathe in and think about what you said as you exhale. It's your choice, but you need to find a program that reliably helps you to relax. Now we return to the states of mind: "Coma," "Sleep," "Awake," "Hyper," and "Relaxation." Remember that one of the features of the awake mind is the ability, the *necessity*, to focus on one thing at a time in the midst of sensory and thought grenade bombardment. Thankfully, this talent comes in handy for people trying to relax. The more you focus on one thing, the more all other sensory and thought "incomings" cannot hit home in your brain. They are still landing in your brain, but they don't explode in a way that disturbs you.

Someone in the group invariably resists the "Focus" imperative with a reminder that their worry and fear thoughts are going to keep on coming, and so is the pain. "Fair enough, so what can you do about that? What if I said, 'My son just called from the police station, and I am going to take 10 calming breaths before I say anything?'" Many group members resist this suggestion that pausing for emotional detachment from such an aggravating or scary event could work, but no one thinks that the ability to do so wouldn't be super helpful in their lives. We are talking about the ability to let go of troubling thoughts before they can explode into suffering. I write "Letting go" on the board.

Now we return to falling asleep. "What position were you in when you fell asleep?" All the sleepers were lying down. When relaxing, it is possible—but less likely—that you will fall asleep if you are sitting, unless you have a rare disorder called narcolepsy. You are not going to fall asleep if you are standing or walking. It may be easier for you to attain relaxation when lying on your back in early attempts, but most people find they get better results and don't fall asleep if they are sitting, standing, or walking. Many people draw a hidden benefit from this realization. The same technique that helps them relax deeply while sitting or standing helps them overcome their problems with insomnia. They just use the same technique lying quietly under the covers at bedtime. Back pain is often aggravated by prolonged sitting, so the traditional lotus or chair sitting may be intolerable. Virtually everyone with chronic back pain can walk, so walking with very slow steps, breathing out with each foot plant and breathing in with each bringing the back foot forward,

| COMA | SLEEP | AWAKE | HYPER |
|---|---|---|---|
| | | Counseling | Adrenaline |
| **RELAXATION** | | $ | **FIGHT/FLIGHT** |
| Quiet | | Family | ^ Breathing |
| Focus | | Spouse/kids | ^ Heart rate |
| Breathing | | Work | ^ Blood pressure |
| Letting go | | Boss/co-workers | |
| Posture | | Sex | ^ Muscles!! |
| | | Sickness | |

**Figure 5.2.**

is manageable and effective. To summarize our discussion of physical positioning and movement, I write "Posture" on the board.

I complete today's board by adding the four key elements of producing the relaxation response: "Quiet," "Focus/Breathing," "Letting go," and "Posture." In reviewing the board shown in figure 5.2, everyone complains that there is no way they can make those things happen in the midst of daily life. They have pain. They have family feuds and TVs blaring or electronic games to wrest from their children. They have noisy neighbors. Their phones are ringing or dinging all the time. They have to cook dinner. The toilet is running. Look at all these bills. On and on goes the list of intrusions. Precisely. Finally, we are ready to look at the list of true stressors in life and how to not let them drive you from "Awake" to "Hyper." Now we can talk about going from "Awake" to "Relaxation" when the crap hits the fan.

## WHY TO RELAX

Money, family feuds, sex, sickness, politics, or worries of any kind can cause so much suffering. Day in and day out—and for some of us all night long—these stressors make us miserable. If there were a pill you could take to quell your emotional response to them so you could face them with a cool mind, wouldn't that be awesome? The group knows all about this "dream," and at least a few members are willing to open up about their efforts to chill under fire. Alcohol and sedating drugs, with or without prescriptions, pervade our culture when it comes to calming our worried minds. Everyone in the FRP group who is brave enough to be honest with the group about their experience with booze or downers reports that whatever numbing of their emotional responses to stressors in their lives they achieved has routinely proven temporary and ineffective in true problem solving. Most people admit that these chemical solutions actually made things worse. The effects of sedation can be as bad or worse than the "Hyper" state and fight-or-flight reaction they were trying to blunt in the first place.

> Robert: "When I was a kid, the best way to hide what was going on at home was to stay away from people. It got so I couldn't deal. I guess that's how I ended up living and working by myself. Sometimes I get the shakes just knowing I have to go to the store. Even coming here and being in the group freaked me out at first. Sorry I was so quiet. No offense."

## PAIN AND RELAXATION

Many FRP group members doubt they can use relaxation as we have discussed it to deal with the life stressors we have listed, but no one denies that they would be better off emotionally if they could. So, we turn to the problem of pain. "What if I told you I have 9/10 pain in my back but it's not bothering me?" We have talked about this hypothetical before, and the group routinely reacts again with disbelief and disdain. "More specifically, what if I were putting the ice cream back in the freezer and felt a wave of my pain shoot through my back and pelvis? Let's say I spend a few minutes slowly walking around the kitchen, paying attention to my breathing with each step and letting thoughts about how my life sucks because of my back pain just pass through my mind and out the window?" Here is how most groups respond to this proposition. They don't believe it, but they wish that it could be true for them. I used to repeat that chronic pain causes suffering only if you give it meaning and that letting go of negative interpretations of pain could bring emotional relief. I gave up on that. Listening to the patients over many years has taught me that you have to experience that kind of relief to believe it can happen for you.

Everyone wishes that relaxation could lessen their suffering, and that is enough for me to encourage them to commit to choosing a relaxation technique and practicing it for 20 minutes once (if not twice) a day for at least the 21 days of their training program. This is the schedule that patients in long-term follow-up report has given them the skill to bring on the relaxation response when they are in pain. These veterans routinely opine that brief exposure in the FRP to a few techniques and a lecture on the history and science of relaxation would have been no help to them if they hadn't done their daily practice routines.

## RELAXATION ROUTINE

I wrap up today's session with this simple prescription:

- Choose a sitting, standing, or walking routine. Focus on your breathing, whether counting or repeating a positive thought.
- Commit to practicing your routine for 20 minutes, one or two times per day, in a quiet place for each of the 21 days in your training program.
- Think of your relaxation routine as a tool in your self-care kit for future episodes of pain. You are going to need it, as you will see in the next chapter on acute and chronic pain.

# · 6 ·

# Acute and Chronic Pain

"You've got to be kidding me! This must be some kind of cosmic joke." These were my first thoughts when I woke up one morning 7 days before I had scheduled myself to start writing this chapter. When I tried to roll out of bed, a sharp pain shot through my lower back into my abdomen. Expletive! I lay there for half an hour trying not to panic as I worked my way over to the side of the bed. I somehow got both feet on the floor, only to realize I couldn't straighten up enough to walk to the bathroom. Finally, I braced my upper body by pushing my hands down on both thighs and hobbled over to the toilet. Moments later, I couldn't turn to wipe myself. Unable to stand, I dropped forward onto my knees and crawled out to the bedroom floor. I lay there in a fetal position for an hour.

"How did I get here?" I would have laughed at the irony of my situation if I hadn't known that laughing, coughing, and sneezing could send jolts of pain through my back. There I was lying on the floor, flattened by the very problem I was supposed to be a world expert in. Before I tell you what I went through to recover from this "back attack," I'll take you briefly through my education on the subject.

When I was in medical school in the 1970s, it was not uncommon to admit an adult with sudden onset back pain to the hospital for several days of strict bed rest. This tradition of resting the painful spine had grown out of the time-honored orthopedic approach to fractures: fix the bone in place with a cast or pins and plates until it is mended. Lying in bed was broken up only by meals and calls for the bedpan. An occasional physical therapy visit combined heat applications with some massage—if you were lucky. In the days approaching discharge, some instruction in bringing your knees up to your chest while remaining on your back progressed to sitting, then standing and walking. Beyond an X-ray, there were no images done unless you had unrelenting leg pain, lost bowel or bladder control, or couldn't move or feel anything in your legs. These potentially dire consequences of nerve damage from a herniated disc or tumor called for a myelogram, which involved injecting dye into your spinal canal and taking X-rays to look for the offending anatomy. Most people did not require imaging, though, and eventually they were discharged from the hospital with a diagnosis of "medical back pain," meaning they had not had surgery. A true anatomic diagnosis was virtually never made.

Through my medical school and internal medicine residency years, computed tomography and magnetic resonance imaging were gradually introduced in hospitals throughout the United States. More and more pathology was thus discovered, particularly including disc herniations and degenerative disc disease, as described in chapter 3. As a result, more and more surgeries were done, and surgeons became the "real" experts on back pain in most medical communities. So grateful for the excellent training I received in my residency, I launched into medical practice primed to care for people with heart attacks, lung disease, cancer, and infections. When it came to the patients who attended my office with back pain, I had to admit I had no clue what to do.

For several months, I committed Thursday nights to reading everything I could get my hands on about back pain. Standard medical and surgical texts joined chiropractic, osteopathic, and a host of lay books and journal articles on my bookshelf. There were so many inconsistencies, even flat-out arguments, about which anatomic spinal "parts" were generating the pain, their biomechanical and physiological processes, and the appropriate treatment. I concluded there was no right answer, no one-size-fits-all to back pain.

During my residency, I had heard about Dr. James Cyriax, a British orthopedic surgeon who devoted his career to nonoperative care of people with painful musculoskeletal disorders. I attended his serial courses over the next few years and learned rudimentary manipulations and injections for back pain and sciatica. I had successes and failures along a steep learning curve, but one pattern emerged with striking clarity. The most commonly effective manual maneuvers involved the patient lying on his stomach while I pressed down on his lower back with my hands. Usually, the relief was temporary, so I began teaching these responders to perform a replica of the manipulation by lying on their stomachs at home and propping their chests up on a pillow. I also passed on to the patients Dr. Cyriax's mantra, "Keep your back hollow." By this, he meant to maintain the forward curve of the lower back, known as lordosis. This is the same curve that is exaggerated by the manipulation and stomach lying I was using, so the mantra made sense to the patients who had responded to my treatment and advice. I had many happy customers, and my practice rapidly swelled with people complaining of back pain.

At this point in the early 1980s, I met Robin McKenzie. A physical therapist from New Zealand, Robin had discovered that he could teach people how to treat their own backs by performing self-care exercises, like being their own chiropractors. Although we had our differences as to the anatomic source of back pain and the impact of psychological stressors, we fundamentally agreed, based on our personal clinical experiences, that most people had a mechanical pattern to their back pain such that simple forward or backward movement and positioning of the spine could be therapeutic. We became fast friends and colleagues. The World Rehabilitation Fund supported my fellowship with Robin, during which we studied the measurement of lordosis in the lower spine, the key direction of relief for most people with back pain. You will find Robin's book *Treat Your Own Back* in the Suggested Readings at the end of this book. Although I don't agree with every word in it, I highly recommend this sensible book to anyone suffering from back pain.

## PHYSICIAN, HEAL THYSELF

Back to my story. Once I got to my feet and made my way out to the kitchen, I saw myself in the mirror and realized I was tilted at the waist off to my right. I tried to straighten up by leaning into a doorjamb, but that was a no-go. It took me 10 long minutes to descend the short staircase to my office in the basement. I looked through my stack of books and articles on back pain. I stifled my laughter over how totally inconsistent and confusing all the thousands of pages of advice were. What to do? Bend forward, bend back, rest, go for a walk, take a muscle relaxant, take an anti-inflammatory, hang upside down, call the chiropractor, get a massage.

Two observations hit me over the head. First, sitting was an absolute no-no. Even when I could manage sitting long enough to eat a meal, I couldn't stand up without a few painful minutes of pushing myself up from the table. Sitting was out for the next few days. I could accommodate that conclusion, but the second sensation was more challenging.

I felt this strange tension spreading through my torso. There was some discomfort deep in my back whenever I was standing or walking, but always at the back of my mind was the command to not make a move that would bring on the excruciating jabs of pain, like someone pounding me in the back with a hammer. This conscious or unconscious protecting of the back is known in medical parlance as "guarding," and I was all too aware that persistent restriction of movement can lead quickly to stiffening and weakening of the structures supporting the spine. "Use it or lose it" came to mind.

This feeling of my back tightening has often been described in medical texts as "spasm," a putative indication for muscle relaxant pills. I reminded myself that this was not a matter of sustained involuntary muscle contraction because I could release it by lying down and taking a few deep breaths. I have never tried muscle relaxants, but I did drink a beer with limited success in relieving what I started calling in my self-talk "spinal anxiety." As the day wore on, so did my worries mount. What was going on in my back? How long would it hurt and lay me up? The same questions my patients had asked me now came on with a vengeance. Through the next few days, I experienced a consequence many patients have reported to me over the years. The physical and mental "work" required to deal with this tension in my back was exhausting.

SELF-TALK

Three bits of knowledge eventually saved the day. First, I had been through this exact scenario four times before, the last attack occurring a few years ago. I had had the same pain in the same place: right at the junction between my spine and my sacrum. I had no leg pain or strength or sensory loss, and my bowel and bladder were working fine. I knew that a recurrence of a familiar pattern of pain virtually never indicated a "serious" underlying cause, namely, cancer. Second, I knew the odds on recovery no matter what I did. My chances of becoming pain free in a matter of days or weeks were excellent. Third, I recalled from prior episodes that a combination of lying on my stomach and propping up my chest with a pillow to create lordosis in my lower back could temporarily relieve my pain and that sitting would make things worse. Anti-inflammatory medication (ibuprofen) seemed to help, so that was worth a try. I knew a call or a visit to a health care facility was unlikely to help, so I committed to a few days of the self-care stretches, ibuprofen, going for walks, and keeping active by writing this chapter with my computer on a chest-high shelf. I went for two or three walks each day. I couldn't put socks on. I found some oversized slippers I could slide into. I developed a blister on my right big toe and had to cover it with a band-aid. Pathetic! I also decided to use a relaxation technique called a "body scan," which you can access by visiting the website https://palousemindfulness .com as listed in the Suggested Readings at the end of this book. I'll let you know how things turned out in the this book's epilogue.

## ACUTE PAIN

Just to make sure we are all on the same page, I begin today's FRP lecture by asking the group to define the word "acute." Members who do not have any medical training invariably think the word means "severe." In contrast, when I ask them what it means to have chronic pain, they all know this term denotes problems that have been going on for a long time. Now they are ready for the medical definitions of acute and chronic pain and the power that understanding these definitions can give to their own self-management of pain.

Acute pain comes on suddenly, with or without trauma. Think of a broken bone or a sprained ankle. The sudden onset is rapidly followed by a period of inflammation. Blood vessels bring cells and chemicals to the wounded tissue, creating heat, redness, swelling, and pain as described in chapter 4. Inflammation also sets up the healing process, including bone and scar formation, depending on which tissue has been injured. This process follows a typical pattern of resolution of pain and return of function over a matter of days and weeks. Medical and surgical providers can comfortably predict that injured patients will recover comfort and get back on their feet in 6 to 8 weeks, sooner in most cases. Most adults have experienced this biological pathway from injury to inflammation to healing to symptomatic resolution and functional recovery.

Chronic pain is a different ball game. Most medical texts on the subject start the clock on chronic pain at about 3 months after onset. After that, the healing process is over. Further spontaneous recovery is not expected anytime soon, maybe not for months or years. The chances of discovering a fixable source of the pain plummet to almost nil. The stiffness, weakness, and loss of endurance born of protective limitation of physical activity make up the deconditioning syndrome described in chapter 1.

I ask the group members to imagine they stepped on a nail. You or a medical provider extract the nail and clean the wound. The site is tender and inflamed, so you walk favoring that foot or use crutches for a while. So far, your pain is acute and likely to resolve as expected. Happy days! But let's say that, for whatever reason, 3 months go by, and your pain has not gone away. Not only does your foot still hurt, but your opposite knee and your back are also aching from the asymmetrical gait you have developed to protect your foot. You have stopped going to the gym, and you notice you are winded going upstairs like never before. You have gained 20 pounds. Your customary cocktail in the evening has turned into four or five starting in the mid-afternoon. And how are you feeling about life at this point? Your doctor can't explain or fix your problem, and your spouse wonders what the hell is wrong with you.

The FRP group members know all about this situation, and they have no problem listing all the psychological stressors and reactions they have experienced for themselves as their own problems progressed past the 3-month deadline. We have discussed their experiences along these lines in previous meetings, so I ask them to hold off on further discussion so that we can move on to the meat of today's class: flare-ups.

## FLARE-UPS

A flare-up is the sudden recurrence or exacerbation of a familiar pattern and quality of pain. It hurts in the same place and feels the same as it has before, whether once or twice in the past year or twice a week for the past few months. A flare-up must be distinguished from sudden onset of a new symptom, such as new leg pain accompanied by loss of strength and/or sensation, which could signal spinal nerve damage. I am confident in telling the FRP groups that the staff are very well trained to evaluate such new pain and getting appropriate help if needed. This is different from the reaction to flare-ups of familiar pain that the patients can expect from the staff. For a brief period in the middle of my experience with FRPs, the staff addressed *all* episodes of pain by stopping the physical exercise and applying heat, massage, and manipulation. Careful review of the outcomes from this period showed that the patients were not making significant gains in flexibility, strength, and endurance. I recalled reports that a separate rehabilitation program had also failed to produce meaningful functional gains while practicing similar acute care practices. The staff retrained to encourage the patients to "use their skills" to combat flare-ups, just as they would have to once discharged back into the "real" world. The patients' physical capacity results improved almost immediately.

By this point in the FRP, every group has described their own experiences with flare-ups, as represented by the graph in figure 1.3. Now we are ready to have a look at their responses to the questionnaire that you see in figure 6.1. If you have had experience with episodes or flare-ups of low back pain, do your best to answer the questions for yourself.

In preparing to write this chapter, I reviewed 184 deidentified "Acute Pain Worksheets" completed by consecutive participants on the first day of their FRPs over the years. I can tell you without hesitation that no two are alike. What hits you between the eyes about their

---

**ACUTE PAIN WORKSHEET**

1. Describe the last time your pain suddenly got worse.
2. Where were you? Who was with you?
3. What thoughts went through your mind about the pain?
4. What did you do about the pain?
5. How well did what you did work?

---

**Figure 6.1.**

responses is that the situations in which people experience sudden flare-ups of pain, the thoughts that go through their heads, what they do about their pain, and how it turns out vary widely. I will do my best to take you through the classroom discussions and distill the common threads that led to success and those that failed. Then you will learn the strategies these folks took away from the FRP in personal packages that worked for them, one by one.

## THE LAST TIME YOUR PAIN GOT WORSE

The worksheet begins by asking you to describe the last time your pain suddenly got much worse. Recall that the FRP participants answering this questionnaire have had their pain problems for months if not years. So, they are describing flare-ups, not first-time episodes of back pain. Of the 184 respondents, 69 did not describe the physical situations in which their pain flared up because nothing they considered "special" had happened. Twenty-eight individuals entered single reports of incidents, such as putting on slippers, tripping, coughing, or getting dressed. One patient was in a motor vehicle accident. Otherwise, there were no reports of trauma. There is much to be learned from the other 87 people who did write in their circumstances:

Performing housework or kitchen work: 22
Sitting in a car: 18
Sitting elsewhere: 16
Lifting: 12
Shopping: 11
Getting out of bed in the morning: 8

What do these activities have in common? They all involve bending forward at the waist. Housework includes sweeping, vacuuming, picking things up off the floor, loading and unloading clothes dryers and washing machines, and cleaning objects and surfaces mostly below the waist. Working at the kitchen counter and cooking appliances requires prolonged periods of bending forward at the waist. In order to sit down, you must rotate your pelvis backward such that your upper body weight ends up in front of your lower spine. Although sitting relieves the big leg muscles from the work of standing, that happens at the expense of creating greater downward force through your spine than standing in a neutral position. Try standing with a 45-degree forward bend at the waist. That position compresses your lower spine with the same amount of force as does sitting. If you have a back problem, you know that staying in that position is not going to feel good.

You might think that lifting predictably fires up low back pain and that the greater the load, the greater the pain. Consider the things the FRP patients reported lifting. A few loads make the grade, like firewood, hay bales, and tree limbs. But the rest of the list—a soda can, a child's toy, a plastic bin, and a hairbrush—make you wonder whether the bending forward wasn't more to blame than the weight of the load. FRP patients claim that shopping brings on back pain when, after prolonged walking bent over a cart, they reach down to get an item off a lower shelf, sit in the changing room, or put a loaded bag into the car. How about getting out of bed in the morning? Where is the trauma there? The movement that strikes up the lower back is trying to raise the upper body, as in a sit-up, using muscles that compress the spine in the same direction and force as sitting and lifting.

Overall, these chronic back pain veterans' responses to the worksheet reveal that flare-ups of back pain come on primarily with some form of everyday loading of the spine in flexion (bending forward at the waist) or with no particular incident or event. Unfortunately, despite Dr. Cyriax's admonition to "keep your back hollow," there is just no way to completely avoid trunk flexion throughout the day given the demands of everyday life. We will capitalize on the "curse of flexion" when we address the fourth question in the "Acute Pain Worksheet": "What did you do about the pain?" First, let's have a look at the FRP patients' responses to the third question.

## YOUR THOUGHTS DETERMINE YOUR ACTIONS

The 184 FRP responders to this questionnaire came up with 202 "thoughts" that went through their heads when their back pain suddenly flared up. I'll summarize them in categories here:

Frustration, anger, and fear: 78
Consequences: 34
Cause: 23
Severity: 21
Duration: 13
Injury: 11
Bravery: 11
Positive action: 11

In frequency and severity, frustration and its cousins, fear and anger, top the list. "I am so sick of this." "Again?" "I hate this stupid, f——ing pain." "Why can't it just stop?" "I just wanted to cry." "Give me a gun. One shot." When you consider how many times people with long-standing back pain suffer through these episodes of severe pain, often without any clear explanation or guarantee of quick relief, it's no wonder they immediately respond to a sudden attack with negative emotions.

Closely related to the fear and frustration, worries about the consequences of the attack rush through the mind. "Does this mean I can never do this thing that I love to do?" "I can't even clean my house." "What if I can't make it back to my car?" "Will I be able to get up the stairs?" "How am I going to take care of the kids?" "What if I can't take care of myself?" "Will I be able to finish the last week of school?" "Do I have to have another operation?" Thoughts about causality run the gamut from annoyance that an act so trivial could cause such terrible pain to wondering exactly what the person did to bring on the attack. Maybe you could avoid the activity if you knew what it was. People often call themselves stupid for doing something that apparently caused their pain only to realize the act was something they have done hundreds of times with impunity.

Expletives commonly told the story of severity, joined by phrases like "I wanted to scream." and "Oh great, now I'm totally screwed." Tied with expressions of pain, immediate questions of duration came up. The question, "Will this never end?" took two forms: "How long will this flare-up last?" and "Will this keep happening for the rest of my life?" The question as to whether this episode represents a recurrence of the same old problem or some new injury involving true tissue damage and possibly the need for medical care must be answered every time. Everyone needs to know how to answer this question for him- or herself, and we will get to that when we put together the personal self-care kit at the end of this chapter.

On a possibly positive note, 11 of the responses reflected the patient's ability to summon courage and push through the pain to accomplish the task at hand. On the other hand, only 11 responses related to taking positive action, such as stretching, moving, relaxing, or applying ice.

Undeniably, the ratio of worries, fears, and frustrations to positive self-talk was overwhelming at 180 to 22. So, let's see what actions the FRP patients took to deal with their flare-ups.


## WHAT TO DO WHEN PAIN STRIKES

The 182 patients employed 282 strategies to combat their acute pain episodes. Here they are, listed in order of frequency:

Medications: 75
Rest, reducing, or stopping activity: 59
Stretching: 34
Ice/heat: 31
Keeping active: 22
Sitting: 16
Nothing: 13
Relaxing: 10
Not sitting: 8
Emergency room care: 8
Redirecting thoughts: 6

You can see that these veterans of chronic pain treated their flare-ups with medications and rest as often as all the other strategies put together. What you can't see is that the severity of the pain and the reported causal event did not appear to determine the choice of treatment. One patient was out for a walk and suddenly had so much pain that she could hardly make it back to her house. She sat on a heating pad, and the pain resolved. The patient who picked up a hairbrush ended up in the emergency room. The situation does matter, though. If your back attacks while you are in the grocery store and your little kids are with you, your immediate options for self-care are different than they would be if you were at home alone or in an out-of-town restaurant with business associates. Considering the questionnaires as a whole, I could not help but notice (as the FRP participants always did when hearing each other's stories) that back pain can come on at any time and in any place.

## WHAT TREATMENT WORKS BEST?

The last question in the worksheet asks, "How well did what you did work?" I graded the responses as best I could from 0, meaning not at all, to 10, meaning complete relief. The results formed a bell-shaped curve with some people doing very well, some doing very poorly, but most having equivocal results. Unfortunately, there were no clear winners on the self-treatment list. This failure to declare a "best treatment" for flare-ups from the questionnaires came as no surprise to me because it reflected what happened when virtually every FRP group discussed their responses together. What worked for one person often struck the next person as ridiculous.

The FRP sessions in which the patients read to each other their responses to the "Acute Pain Worksheet" always came to a very uncomfortable moment when the group realized these key features of back pain flare-ups:

Flare-ups can happen at any time and in any place.
Triggering events can be trivial, and they are impossible to predict.
There is no single right treatment for everyone.

These observations are disheartening to every FRP group because they imply that flare-ups are not preventable and that treatment is ineffective. These conclusions frequently drive the group to look to me for answers. What can be done? The urgency of this question is all the more pressing when the group recalls how the fear of sudden pain episodes governs their decisions about whether to be active. Some groups practically beg me to tell them what they should do.

I ask the group, "What is the best way to deal with your fear of some event you know will happen in the future but you don't know when or where?" Everyone knows the answer has something to do with being prepared to respond, to having a plan. At this point, I bring up the image of a tool kit. I ask the group members to imagine that they each have a personalized kit available at any time and in any place. In the kit, they have tools they know can be helpful in dealing with a sudden attack of pain. Over the years of caring for people with chronic pain and listening to what has worked for FRP graduates, I feel very confident in telling the current group what their predecessors have put into their tool kits. They already know from listening to each other that there is no right treatment for all, so it is not hard to understand that they must figure out which tools to put into their personal kits for themselves.

I go to the whiteboard and write out the key tools for flare-ups, as you can see in figure 6.2:

---

**FLARE-UP TOOL KIT**

Relaxation/Breathing

Positive thoughts

Physical self-care

Medication

Movement

---

**Figure 6.2.**

Relaxation/breathing: Now is the time to call up the calming, peaceful state of mind you have made your own by practicing whatever relaxation technique you have chosen. For most people, a method of measured breathing is most practical in the midst of an acute pain attack since it can be done standing, walking, or lying down. That makes it possible to perform no matter what your situation may be when your back acts up. Your mind is much more open to the next step if it is calm.

Positive thoughts: Ask yourself if this pain is something new or whether it is a recurrence or flare-up of the same old problem. Does it hurt in a new place, or is there a new loss of sensation or strength in your leg? Did you lose control of your bowel or bladder? If not, and you recognize this pain as your usual pain, proceed.

Physical self-care: Keep it simple. You can lie down, sit, or stand, and you can bend forward or backward at the waist or twist to right or left in either posture. The best way to find out what works for you is to try different approaches to reduce your pain when it is not too bad. The movement or posture that relieves your usual pattern of pain is known in medical circles as your "directional preference." A skilled physical therapist or chiropractor can help you find your preference in a visit or two if you have one. You may be able to discover your personal relief regimen for yourself in Robin McKenzie's book *Treat Your Own Back*, listed in the Suggested Readings at the end of this book.

Medication: Keep handy an emergency supply of whatever medication(s) you and your doctor have arrived at for acute pain treatment as described in chapter 4.

Movement: If you can't move, you can't move. As soon as you can manage it, though, gently progressive movement is the key. Start walking, even if you have to start with small, slow steps, wherever you are. If you have to lie down, get up as soon as you can. Avoid sitting at all costs.

These are the fundamental tools that, year after year, people have told me worked best for them. But you must find the tools that work for *you*. I recommend to each member of the group that they write down their list of tools and keep a copy of the list on their nightstand, in the kitchen, in their car, at their workstation, or wherever they think they might get into trouble. Some people keep a copy in their wallet or purse. The most powerful effect of having a plan you have worked on and believe in comes from reducing whatever fear you may have of your next flare-up and from the freedom that courage brings you to lead an active life.

Speaking of an active life, the group is now ready to talk about wellness, the subject of chapter 7.

## • 7 •

# Wellness

$\mathcal{E}$ach month, the functional restoration program (FRP) session on wellness was my last opportunity to meet with the patients as a group. For some people, this was the most important of all our meetings. For most people, especially in the formative years of the discussion, the session was a complete waste of time. In those early days, the discussion was actually a lecture on the importance of a healthy diet. We also came down pretty heavily against cigarette smoking.

No doubt, the smoking cessation made generic sense as a strategy for reducing the patients' risk of heart disease and cancer. Of course, everyone already knew that. However, it came as news to all that smoking also increased your chances of having back pain, presumably by reducing blood flow to your spine. Ironically, we gave up on encouraging people to stop smoking while they were in the program. They had enough on their hands just coping with pain and the challenges of progressive exercise, being away from home, and making plans for their futures. Quitting smoking was one stressor we could eliminate for the time being.

Diet was a different deal. The lecture laid out what was known as the food pyramid. The "teacher" led the group through the layers from the "good for you" foods on the bottom to the killer foods on the top. Patient responses ranged from outright contention from patients who had their own contradictory beliefs about nutrition to the majority reaction: nap time. Over the years, the staff made two observations that turned the tables. First, the food pyramid began to crumble with uncertainties from the experts as to what we "should" be eating and how much of each of the different food groups. More important, the patients

## GRETA

Greta sits on your left today. You have avoided sitting next to her because she always smells like she just smoked a cigarette. During the group walk yesterday, you found her to be a truly nice person, though. You were surprised to find that, in contrast with her heaviness and rough southern slang, she is a nurse turned massage therapist. You wonder how someone who is in a caring profession could be so sloppy about taking care of herself. She did tell you that she grew up in a foster home without much attention from her parents. She worked her way through nursing school, but too much hospital sickness and death got to her. She knows massages don't necessarily cure diseases, but she really connects with her clients, and they love her. "My life took a dive in the toilet, Honey," she says about losing her job when her back hurt too much to bend forward long enough to perform table massages.

just did not see how what they ate made any difference to their chief complaints of low back pain.

Occasionally, someone would ask whether dietary supplements and vitamins could reduce their pain. Chondroitin sulfate and glucosamine had a champion or two but without enough evidence for the lecturer to advise the group one way or the other. Finally, we gave up on the nutrition lecture. We realized we didn't really know what we were talking about in the context of chronic pain, and the patient satisfaction ratings were dismal.

Just as with the sessions on goals, drugs, and doctor visits, the inspiration for the wellness discussion came from listening to the patients. Beyond achieving their goals as described in chapter 2, they wanted to know what it would take to get their lives "back together again." For some people, this quest was simply a matter of reverting to the life they had led before they developed back pain. Others were just longing for a happier, more rewarding life than the limited existence they had endured due to their disability.

## HEALTH

"Would you settle for being healthy?" "What would that be like?" I began several final FRP sessions with these questions. Each group responded with their own question: "What do you mean by healthy?" Each patient seemed to have a different definition, but all of them felt it had something to do with not being sick. By being sick, they meant having symptoms like pain, nausea, vomiting, diarrhea, rashes, swollen joints, and so forth. Some people said you couldn't be healthy if you had any diseases like diabetes or hypertension, even if they weren't causing any symptoms. Rarely, a brave soul or two wished out loud for an end to their depression or anxiety. Overall, the groups arrived at the conclusion that health was the absence of symptoms and disease.

Many FRP participants with chief complaints of back pain had comorbidities including hypertension, diabetes, joint pain, cardiac problems, and mood and thought disorders. I asked them if they would be satisfied should they continue with their back pain as is but be able to get rid of their other health problems, whether physical or mental. While everyone wanted their other health problems to go away, especially their pain, many people felt there must be "more to life" than just not being sick or in pain. This "feeling" came up often enough to prompt me to ask the groups about their impressions of wellness.

Greta: "I just wish I wasn't so frickin' fat, is all. Maybe if there was a little less of me, I wouldn't jump for joy all day and stuff, but I don't like what I see in the mirror, for damn sure. Now that I'm home all the time, I look even worse."

"What does wellness mean?" My question was met so routinely by blank stares and silence and responded to so vaguely when there were responses that I gave up on that approach. People seemed to have a general sense that wellness was probably a good thing, possibly more positive in some ways than health. They just couldn't define wellness in any practical way that could guide the group toward a discussion of how to achieve it.

In frustration one day, I blurted out, "Okay, how about death? Anybody looking forward to death?" That caught everyone's attention.

They all agreed that if you were dead, you were not well. As facetious as this conclusion was, it led to a way of talking about wellness that profoundly affected many FRP patients' lives.

## WHAT DO AMERICANS DIE FROM?

Welcome to today's meeting. The people sitting around the table with you now know each other in uncommon ways. That is, they know each other's stories and how back pain destroyed their lives as they were. Maybe their lives weren't perfect before back pain took over. Whatever! Let's talk about *death*.

I step up to the whiteboard and ask the group to call out the most common causes of death in the United States. I write them down along the right side of the board, as you can see in figure 7.1. Everyone knows that heart disease tops the list. I clarify that the leading culprit under the heading of heart disease is "hardening" of the little arteries that feed the heart muscle itself. This is the underlying process that sets

| | | |
|---|---|---|
| Don't smoke | Genes | Heart disease |
| Check/control BP | Hypertension | Cancer |
| Exercise | Obesity/Diabetes | Accidents |
| Don't eat too much | Depression/anxiety | Lung disease |
| Don't drink too much | Alcohol | Stroke |
| Relax | (Insomnia) | Alzheimer's |
| Connect | | Diabetes |
| | | Flu/pneumonia |
| | | Kidney failure |
| | | Suicide |

**Figure 7.1.**

the scene for sudden blocking of the artery and damage or death of the blood-starved heart muscle. Second on the list is cancer, and the top types of cancers that kill are lung, colon, breast, and pancreatic. "We are halfway done." I explain that heart disease and cancer account for more than half of American deaths every year. Accidents are number three on the death list. The fourth is no accident because cigarette smoking is so commonly the cause. Not counting infections, respiratory disease in the form of chronic obstructive pulmonary disease (COPD) kills about 40,000 Americans per year, about the same number that succumb to accidents and stroke. The top 10 killer list is completed with diabetes, influenza/pneumonia, kidney disease, and suicide. The very mention of suicide raises an emotional flag with every FRP group.

## KILLER CONDITIONS

Returning to the board, I ask the group to tell me what health factors or conditions put us at risk for these causes of death. "Bad luck." By this, they mean that the genes you are born with have a lot to do with when and from what you will die. They also mean that accidents can happen to you out of the blue by no fault of your own. Everyone agrees that your genes and most accidents are beyond your control, so I encourage the group to move on to conditions they *can* do something to prevent. Look at the middle column in figure 7.1.

"Stop smoking!" Everyone knows that smoking is bad for you, but now we have a cogent way of making this admonition stick. I draw lines to connect smoking to the diseases we have listed on the right. Heart disease, cancer, and lung disease make three out of the top five. So, "Don't smoke" tops the list of things you can do to prevent death, as you can see in figure 7.1.

> Greta: "Well I don't even know my parents, so the gene thing is out. I learned how to smoke in nursing school. When things got tough in the hospital, we'd go on break and smoke. I really liked that. We were close, you know? My boss smokes, too. It gives us time to chat. I live alone, you know."

## WHAT YOU *CAN* DO

"Control your blood pressure." Hypertension, the silent killer, critically elevates your risk of heart attack and stroke. Everyone in the group knows this, but there is often a debate as to whether you can tell your blood pressure is too high by how you feel. Many people believe they can tell when their blood pressure is high if they are tense or have a headache. I sit down and look these people in the eye. The only practical way to know your blood pressure is to measure it with arm compression and a stethoscope or electronic monitoring device like you see in the doctor's office or pharmacy. So, I write "Check/control BP" (blood pressure) under "Don't smoke." Many people in the FRP program are already taking antihypertensive medications, and the staff carefully measure blood pressures on the day of admission. Normal blood pressure is a critical prerequisite for entry into the exercise program, as it should be for any such endeavor.

"Speaking of exercise, how about getting your heart rate up every day as a means of controlling your blood pressure?" Virtually every patient who has hypertension has already been told that they should exercise, and many have been told to lose weight. I add obesity to the risky conditions list, connecting it to heart disease, cancer, and stroke. I add "Exercise" to the list of preventive actions. What kind of exercise and how much should they do? Although there are formulas for so-called target heart rates, many of the patients who have been disabled by their back pain are starting out far below "normal." Besides, they have already set goals for exercise as part of their admission process, and they have been working on "big muscle" exercise toward these goals on either a treadmill or an exercise bike. By now, they have a pretty clear idea of how much their daily program entails going forward. The lesson to be learned from their experience is to start at a level of walking, biking, or running that is easy for you and build up from there gradually through your 21-day program. Beyond achieving your goals, a reasonable regimen for prevention would be getting your heart rate up to a comfortable level *for you* for at least half an hour per day most days of the week. I recommend you discuss this with your doctor. I frequently recommend reading *Younger Next Year* by Chris Crowley and Henry S. Lodge, MD, as listed in the Suggested Readings at the end of this book.

Greta: "Before my back went out on me, I watched TV a lot. I got into those hot miniseries, you know. Now I can't sit through a show. I tried going to a gym at night a few times. I quit. Too many Lycra babes. I felt like crap there."

"What other conditions and diseases can exercise combat?" Looking at the list of killers on the right, most groups recognize that depression is often the route to suicide. They have also found during their FRP program that heartbeat-raising exercise has lifted their spirits. Month after month, this mood benefit has been documented by impressive improvements in depression questionnaire scores the patients complete before and after the program. Not so obvious is the potential benefit of exercise for people challenged by anxiety and cognitive deficits. For people who are interested in pursuing the mental boons of exercise, I recommend reading John J. Ratey MD's book *Spark*, listed in the Suggested Readings at the end of this book.

We return to the list of risky conditions, and I ask the group what can be done about obesity. We already have "Exercise" on the board. Every group has a short debate about best diets before coming to the same conclusion. I add "Don't eat too much" to the list of preventive actions on the left. Some patients have set goals for weight loss, and I remind them that now is not the time for special diets. When you are focusing on a new regimen of gradually progressive exercise, it makes sense to hold off on changing diet, medication, and even smoking until you have reached your "steady state" of exercise.

Greta: "Look, don't talk to me about food. Food and cigarettes are like my only buddies now. They kinda keep me company, you know?"

## ALCOHOL

I realize we haven't covered one way of preventing killer number three: accidents. When I ask the group for the best way to avoid accidents, they always have the answer. I write "Don't drink too much" (and drive) on the board. In addition to connecting this dictum to accidents, I remind the group that excessive alcohol also increases their risk for hypertension and cancer. "How much is too much?" The easiest answer for an individual goes back to that person's goals. How much alcohol consumption affects your daily functioning in work, recreation, and daily life varies from person to person. I ask the group to consider their goals and be honest about their alcohol consumption in that context. Is booze going to block you from being able to do what matters to you? Someone in the group usually brings up the recent observation that some alcohol appears to prevent cardiac death to some degree. I confirm the recommendation of daily doses of one alcoholic beverage for women and two for men with the caveat that more than that raises the risk flag again. You are better off abstaining if you can't stick with the recommended limits. Again, I recommend *Younger Next Year* for a thoughtful and entertaining read on this subject.

But wait. There is a gaping omission on the board. What can you do that has a track record for reducing the risky conditions of hypertension, anxiety, and depression? Responding to the group's "Aha!," I write "Relax" in the left column. I remind them that insomnia further shortens life—all the more reason to use their relaxation techniques to bring on a good night's sleep. I encourage the group to commit to a daily practice of their chosen relaxation technique for at least 20 minutes through the next few weeks of their training regimen and beyond. Usually by now, the session is nearly over. Before we address the last and most important topic, I recommend to those who want to read more about relaxation Herbert Benson MD's book *The Relaxation Response,* listed in the Suggested Readings at the end this book.

> Greta: "You know, I kinda surprised myself with that walking and breathing thing yesterday. I tried Transcendental Meditation a long time ago. Weird, man. Got to admit, though. If breathing can perk me up and chill me out, I'm in."

## THE MEANING OF *YOUR* LIFE

By the end of the program, I have had a chance to meet with each of the patients a few times individually and witnessed their involvement in the group discussions. Almost everyone has entrusted me with stories of how their back pain has affected their lives. You can appreciate the depth of their concerns by reviewing the previous chapters. There is one theme that runs through virtually everyone's tale of disabling pain: it took me several years of listening to realize that people whose pain restricts the physical activities their previous lives demanded become *disconnected*. They become disconnected from the people and pursuits that gave their life meaning. Disabling pain challenges and often destroys marital and family ties. Friends vanish, especially the ones with whom you shared physical activities you can no longer manage. The sense of self-worth that comes from work and the self-respect that derives from and even depends on boss and coworker acknowledgment both dwindle and die when pain takes away your job.

When it is time for me to say good-bye to the group, I do not bring up these painful stories. I don't need to because each member has already shared their stories with the others. Instead, I stand up and walk back to the board. I write "Connect" at the bottom of the to-do list.

Everyone knows what I mean.

I wish everyone the best of luck with their remaining days in the program and encourage everyone to write down the list of things they can do to live longer and better lives. Here is the formula for wellness:

Check/control blood pressure (BP)
Don't smoke
Exercise
Don't eat too much
Don't drink too much (and drive)
Relax
Connect

# Epilogue

$\mathcal{T}$he characters introduced to you throughout *Talking Back* are mosaics of real participants in functional restoration programs (FRPs) spanning 30 years. Each biographical sketch in the book draws from several individuals, so there is no chance that you will recognize any real person. Here is what happened to each of the "assembled" characters.

## ROBERTA

Roberta had set two top goals for herself. She wanted to get back to work as soon as possible so she could take care of her kids. She also wanted to get back to the gym, her home away from home. She worked hard in the FRP. She didn't get much out of the lectures, and relaxation did nothing for her. Her gains in flexibility and lifting strength were impressive to the staff, but what made all the difference to *her* was her ability to run on the treadmill. That translated into a new aerobic program of jogging and biking. She joined a running club. A newfound friend at the gym introduced her to a travel agent. Her background in finance and the return of the zip in her step won her a job planning walking tours in Europe. When she returned to my office for her 6-month follow-up visit, I hardly recognized her. It's amazing how a smile and laughter can change a person. Her little son was with her. He gave me a card that said, "Thank you for giving me back my mother."

## EDDIE

Eddie made steady progress in the FRP, but rib cage pain kept him from bending forward and turning his trunk enough to manage shoving tree branches into a wood chipper, and his lifting capacity was not good enough to haul logs out of the woods. After graduating from the FRP, he signed up for an adult reading course, thinking he could live with his father and help run the family firewood business. He was going to a local gym every day and maintaining the physical gains he had made in the FRP. Then his attorney called to say his case was settled for more money than Eddie had ever dreamed of. A friend came by to celebrate, and they got drunk, then started shooting up the next day. He could now afford a habit. A few months later, they found Eddie under a bridge. His needle kit was in his coat pocket.

## FRANK

Frank really struggled through the first week of the FRP, especially with the lectures that seemed so anti-doctor. As the other patients asked him to talk about what it was like to be an oral surgeon, they realized together that fixing acutely painful problems had been a wonderful life mission and that he had served his patients well. They also recognized that pain-relieving procedures, like what Frank did every day, could not solve his own problems or theirs. He flushed his remaining Vicodins down the toilet and resolved to stick with his FRP training graphs. His wife attended his FRP graduation and found a new man, like the one she remembered from years ago. He seemed somehow less rigid and more at peace with himself. She wept softly in front of the staff, saying, "I don't know what happened here, but it's like the lights came back on inside him." A year later, Frank sent the FRP staff a photograph and wrote on the back, "Here is a picture of me on Mt. Washington. I hiked it myself. So grateful for the life I got back by lifting those damn milk crates. Thank you."

## WESLEY

No one worked harder than Wesley, and he took every suggestion and piece of advice as an order. His sole goal for the FRP program was to return to military duty. Fortunately, the physical requirements for his duty were clearly delineated in forms forwarded by his medical officer. Running challenged Wesley the most because of his unsteadiness. He stuck with his program of increasing his treadmill work each day. He made it. A few months later, he sent us a picture of his unit. There he was, back in action, serving his country.

## ROBERT

Robert did not achieve his goal of returning to roofing, at least not in the way he had imagined. He did have sufficient physical capacity, as objectively proven by his lifting and treadmill tests. His victory surprisingly came from his success with a relaxation technique he found for himself by combining progressive muscle contraction and relaxation with conscious breathing. He never did overcome his fear of getting back on a roof. He did win his battle with social anxieties by using his relaxation drill when he was stressed around other people. This newfound skill enabled him to work closely with others. He put together his own roofing company. He turned out to be a respected boss, all the more so because he became a key member of his crew, bending metal sheets on the ground.

## MYSELF

Even though I knew all the "tricks of the trade," I reverted to just a few strategies that had helped me get through previous episodes of pain. For the first few days, all I could do was try to adjust my back by lying on my belly with a pillow under my chest and go for walks. I tried ibuprofen, but it upset my stomach. A few times a day, I did a 20-minute meditation routine focusing on my in breath, then my out breath. I woke up every morning dreading the effort to get out of bed. Sitting was the worst. Then the COVID-19 virus struck the United States, and the order to shelter in place came out. I took some of my own medicine. I asked myself what I hoped to accomplish before I died, realizing that my age and cardiovascular troubles put me at risk. I thought about all the people who had participated in FRPs and in the sessions described in this book. I owed it to them, to my colleagues, and *to myself* to complete the book.

So, I set a goal of finishing *Talking Back*. I put together a standing desk, and I dedicated my days to the mission.

My backache improved somewhat over the next month, but one night, I woke up with pain shooting down the back of my left leg into my foot. Oh no! Sciatica. And what if this nighttime onset of new pain heralded cancer? By the next morning, my foot was numb and made a slapping sound as I walked: sure signs of a spinal nerve being compressed. I could just see my MRI showing a herniated disc or a synovial cyst pinching off my fifth lumbar nerve root. My mind spun with fears of injections and surgeries, never to walk right again.

Time for more of my own medicine. I heard myself reassuring hundreds of patients in their throes of sciatica, that their chances of recovery with or without treatment were excellent.

I restarted the ibuprofen three times a day and made myself go for walks at least twice a day. I am so grateful to all the patients who hung in there through their pain and gave me reason to believe my own recitations about spontaneous recovery. Two months along now, I am happy to say I can put on my socks and play golf with no pain and just an occasional feeling that a little ant is crawling up my calf.


## GRETA


The session on going to see the doctor upset Greta, though she kept quiet at the time. As a massage therapist, she had been trained to believe that back pain was a purely muscular matter. So, the failure of differential diagnosis and the subsequent absence of a clear anatomic source for most people with chronic back pain challenged that belief. Her primary goal was to get back to her job as a masseuse, and for that, she needed to tolerate hours of bending forward at the waist. The FRP focus on gradually improving trunk bending and lifting was quickly successful in achieving her work goal. When she returned for her 3-month follow-up, she was accompanied by a very sweet 6-year-old girl: Greta's new foster child. Her camaraderie in the FRP group and her return to her clients had reminded her how important connecting with other people was to her. As soon as her work income allowed it, she qualified to become a foster parent. She didn't have to tell me about the joy these relationships had brought her. You could see it in her eyes.

# Appendix A

**WORKSHEET**

**MEDICAL CLEARANCE QUESTIONS**
for you to answer with your doctor:

Do I have cancer, an infection, a fracture,
or any serious disease that requires treatment?          ___yes ___no

Do I have a structural spinal problem
that requires surgery?          ___yes ___no

Do I have a medical reason not to exercise?          ___yes ___no


**YOUR 4-MONTH GOALS**

PHYSICAL REQUIREMENTS

FLEXIBILITY    STRENGTH    ENDURANCE

WORK


RECREATION


DAILY ACTIVITIES

# Appendix B

## TRAINING CHART

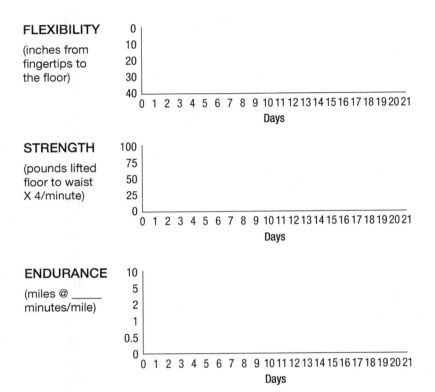

**FLEXIBILITY**

(inches from
fingertips to
the floor)

0
10
20
30
40

0 1 2 3 4 5 6 7 8 9 10 11 12 13 14 15 16 17 18 19 20 21

**Days**

**STRENGTH**

(pounds lifted
floor to waist
X 4/minute)

100
75
50
25
0

0 1 2 3 4 5 6 7 8 9 10 11 12 13 14 15 16 17 18 19 20 21

**Days**

**ENDURANCE**

(miles @ _____
minutes/mile)

10
5
2
1
0.5
0

0 1 2 3 4 5 6 7 8 9 10 11 12 13 14 15 16 17 18 19 20 21

**Days**

# Suggested Readings

## GENERAL BOOKS ON BACK PAIN

Deyo, Richard R. *Watch Your Back! How the Back Pain Industry Is Costing Us More and Giving Us Less*. Ithaca, NY: Cornell University Press, 2014.

Ramin, Cathryn J. *Crooked: Outwitting the Back Pain Industry and Getting on the Road to Recovery*. New York: HarperCollins, 2017.

Waddell, Gordon. *The Back Pain Revolution*. Edinburgh: Churchill Livingstone, 1998.

## SELF-HELP RESOURCES

Benson, Herbert. *The Relaxation Response*. New York: Avon, 1975.

McKenzie, Robin. *Treat Your Own Back*. Raumati Beach: Spinal Publications New Zealand, 2011.

http://www.palousemindfulness.com.

## BOOKS ON THE BENEFITS OF EXERCISE

Crowley, Chris, and Henry S. Lodge. *Younger Next Year: Live Strong, Fit, and Sexy—Until You're 80 and Beyond*. New York: Workman, 2004.

Ratey, John J. *Spark: The Revolutionary New Science of Exercise and the Brain*. New York: Little, Brown, 2008.

## SELECTED PUBLICATIONS
## BY ROWLAND G. HAZARD, MD

Hazard, Rowland G. "Low-Back and Neck Pain: Diagnosis and Treatment." *American Journal of Physical Medicine and Rehabilitation* 86 (2007): 559–68.

———. "Goal Achievement Model for Low Back Pain." *Spine* 38 (2013): 1431–35.

Hazard, Rowland G., et al. "Chronic Low Back Pain: The Relationship between Patient Satisfaction and Pain, Impairment and Disability Outcomes." *Spine* 19 (1994): 881–87.

———. "The Impact of Personal Functional Goal Achievement on Patient Satisfaction with Progress One Year Following Completion of a Functional Restoration Program for Chronic Disabling Spinal Disorders." *Spine* 34 (2009): 2797–2802.

———. "Patient-Centered Evaluation of Outcomes from Rehabilitation for Chronic Disabling Spinal Disorders: The Impact of Personal Goal Achievement on Patient Satisfaction." *Spine Journal* 12 (2012): 1132–37.

# Index

# About the Author

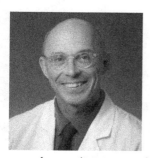

**Rowland G. Hazard**, MD, recently retired from a 30-plus-year career devoted to people disabled by chronic back pain. Currently Emeritus Professor of Orthopaedics at the Geisel School of Medicine at Dartmouth, he is a physician, internationally respected scholar and researcher, widely published author, teacher, inventor, entrepreneur, athlete, and jazz musician.

As a clinician and director of functional restoration programs (FRPs) at the University of Vermont (1986–2000) and at the Dartmouth-Hitchcock Medical Center (2002–2018), Dr. Hazard cared for several thousand patients with back pain and led FRP teams of physicians, psychologists, physical and occupational therapists, and trainers. A board-certified internist, he is a fellow in the American College of Physicians.

He has published more than 50 journal articles and book chapters and delivered scores of related academic lectures and media appearances in the United States, Europe, and Australia. He has served as reviewer and technical expert for the Agency for Healthcare Research and Quality. A reviewer for several medical journals, Dr. Hazard sits on the editorial boards of *Spine* and *The Back Letter*. Elected to membership in the International Society for the Study of the Lumbar Spine in 1988, he has twice served as U.S. representative to the Executive Council. Dr. Hazard lives in Vermont near the farm where he grew up.

Please send comments and suggestions for *Talking Back* to
rowlandhazardmd@gmail.com.

149